MOZAIC
James Douglas Layton
England

"Calm down and color"

Scan this with your
phone to win a free book!!

www.jamesdouglaslayton.com

Instructions:

1: Buy some nice pencils, gell pens or crayons.

2: Grab a chair or hit the sofa.

3: Pour a drink, wine if you can, soda if you like.

4: Get your favorite coloring book.

5: Put a blank sheet of paper under the picture you want to color.

6: Color in the picture.

7: Feel free to cut them out and post them strategically at work to piss off the boss.

P.S - Take a photo and show us, we will show the world your skills.

Calm alone time is your right as an adult. The more relaxed you become the better your life gets.

That's scientific fact!!!

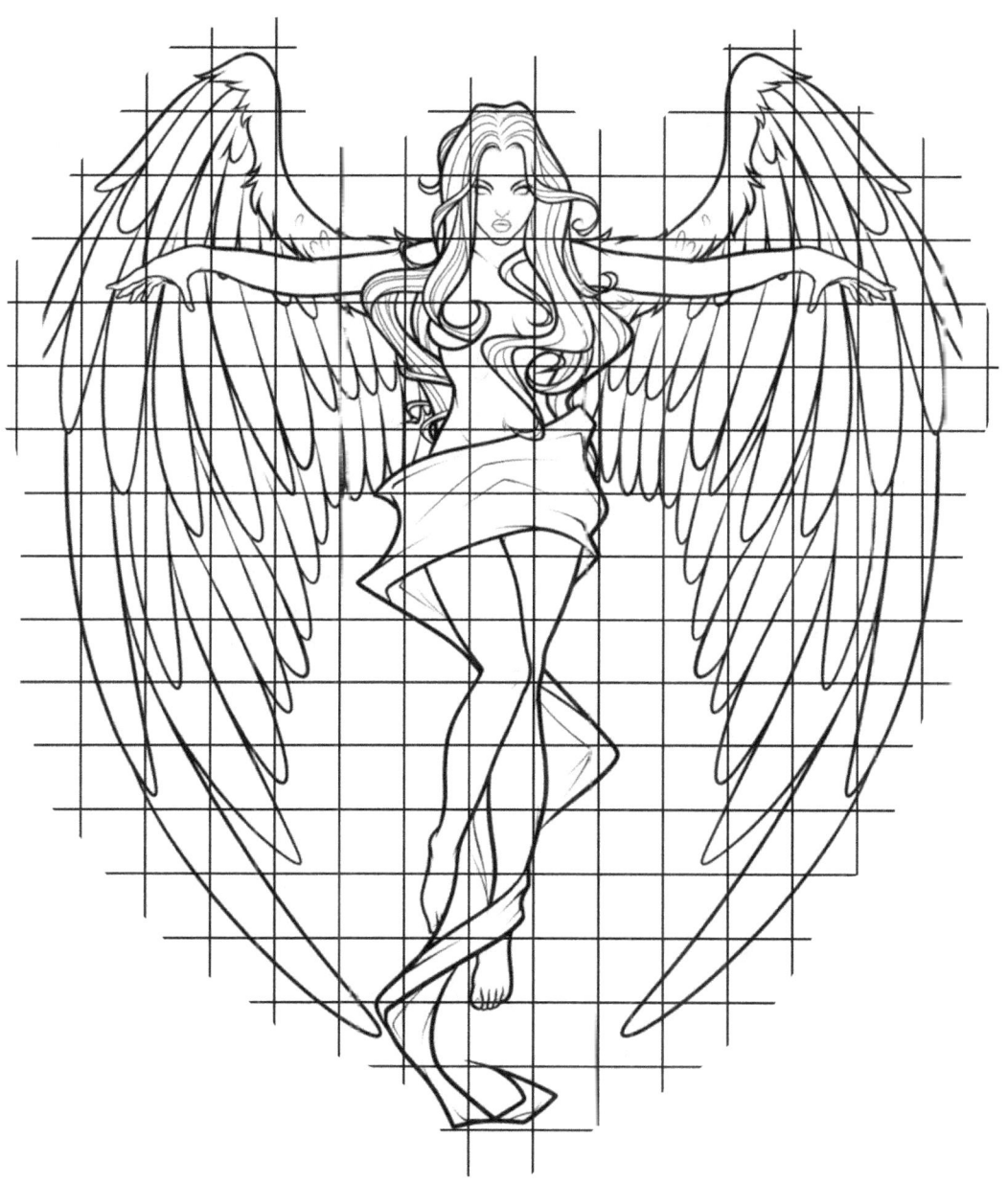

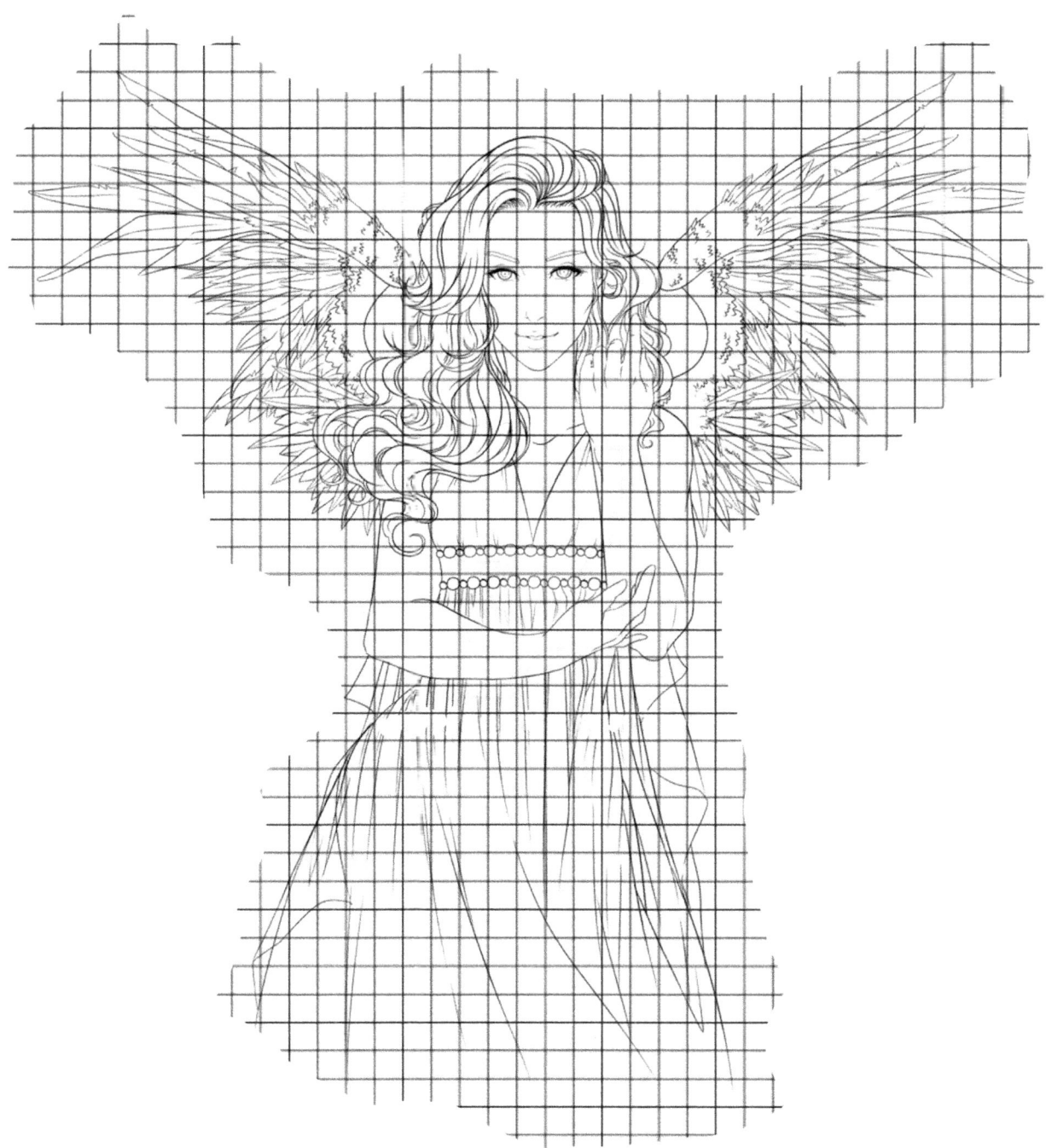

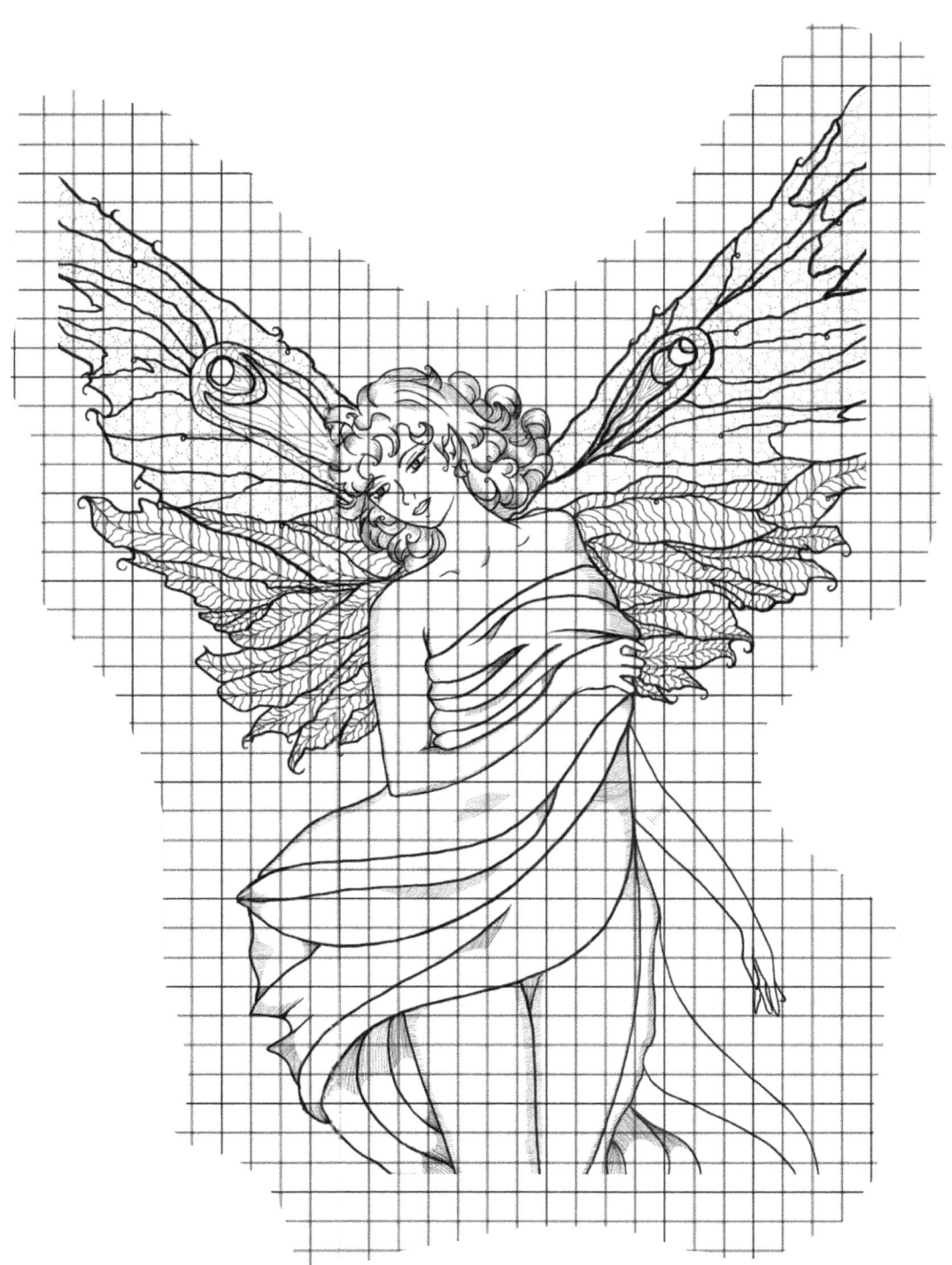

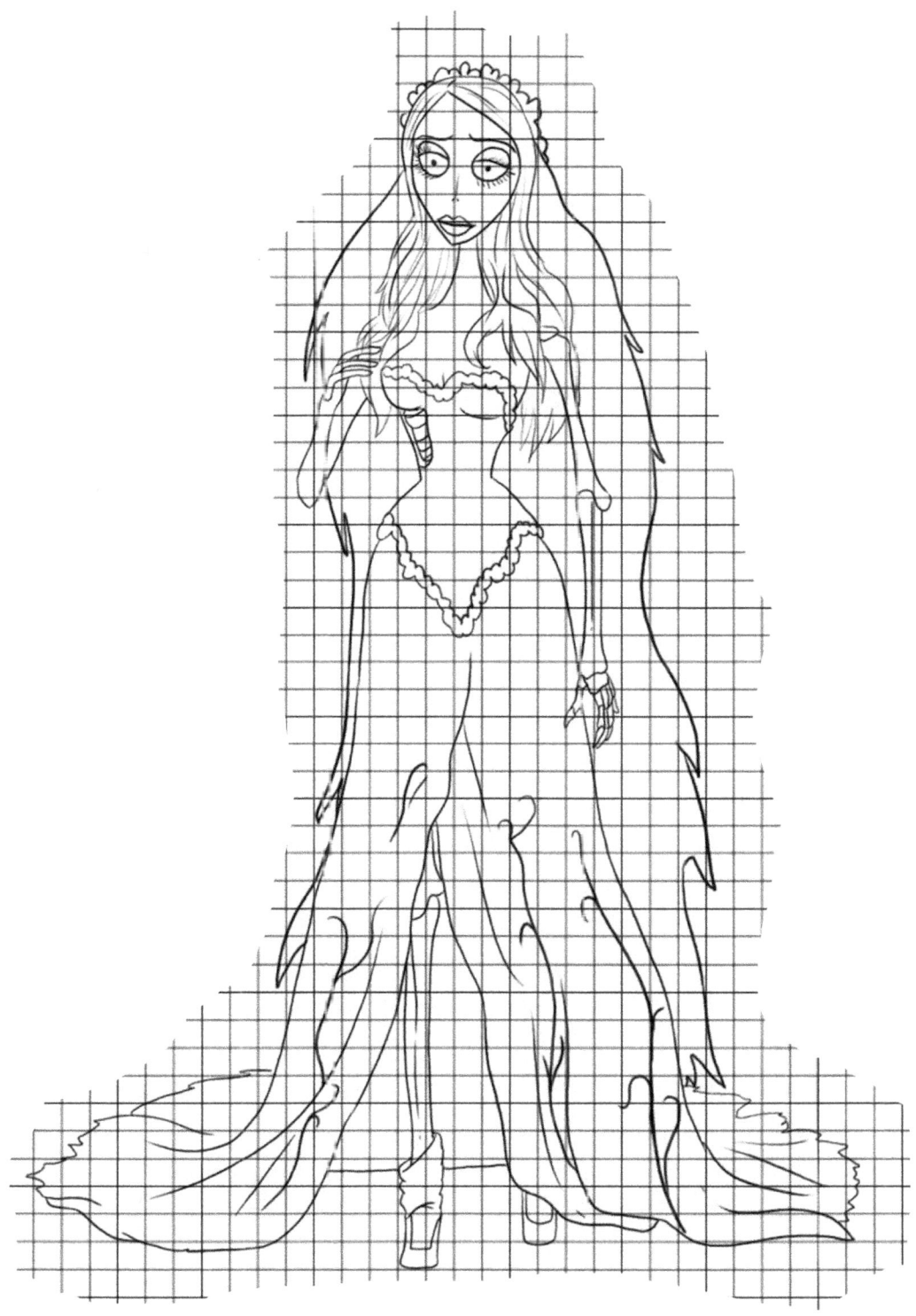

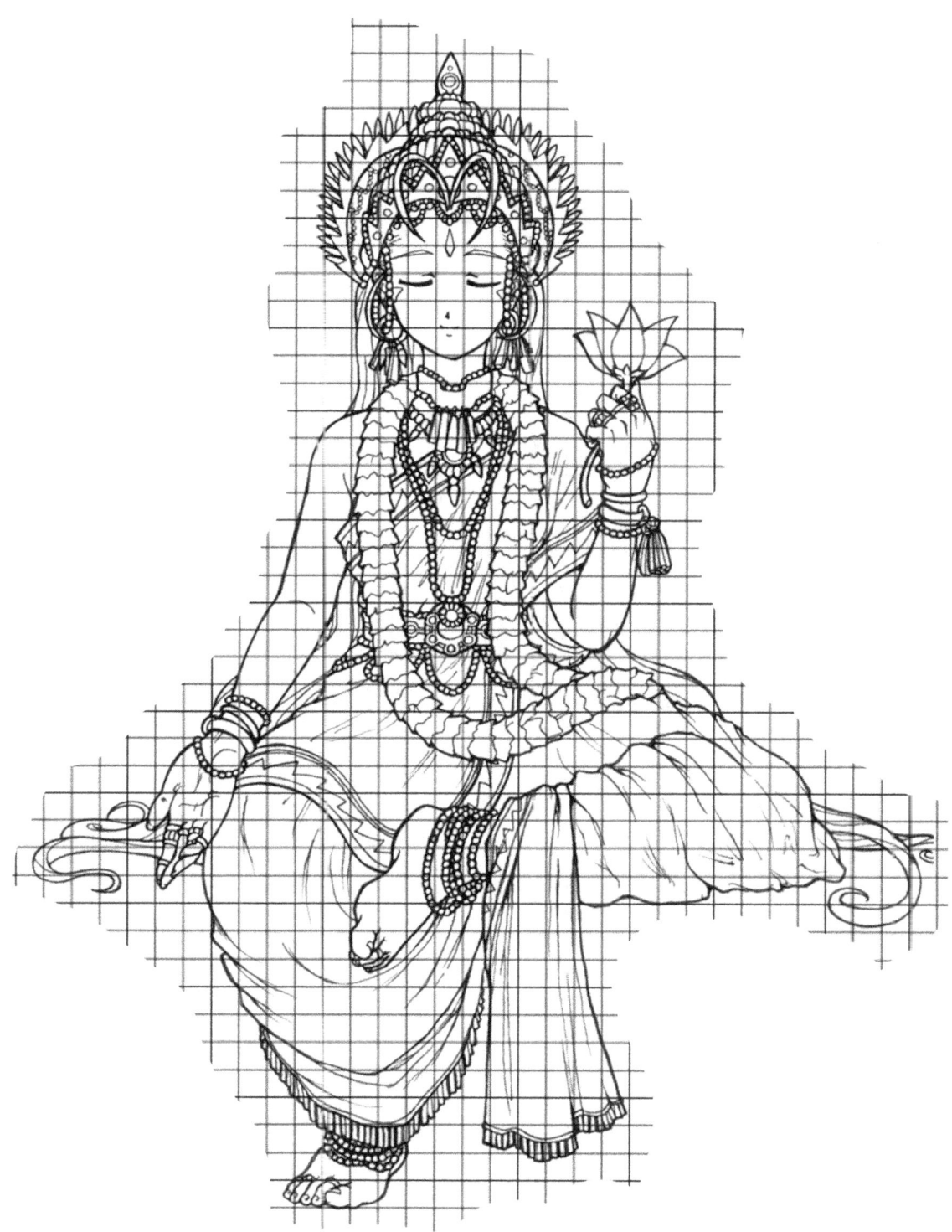

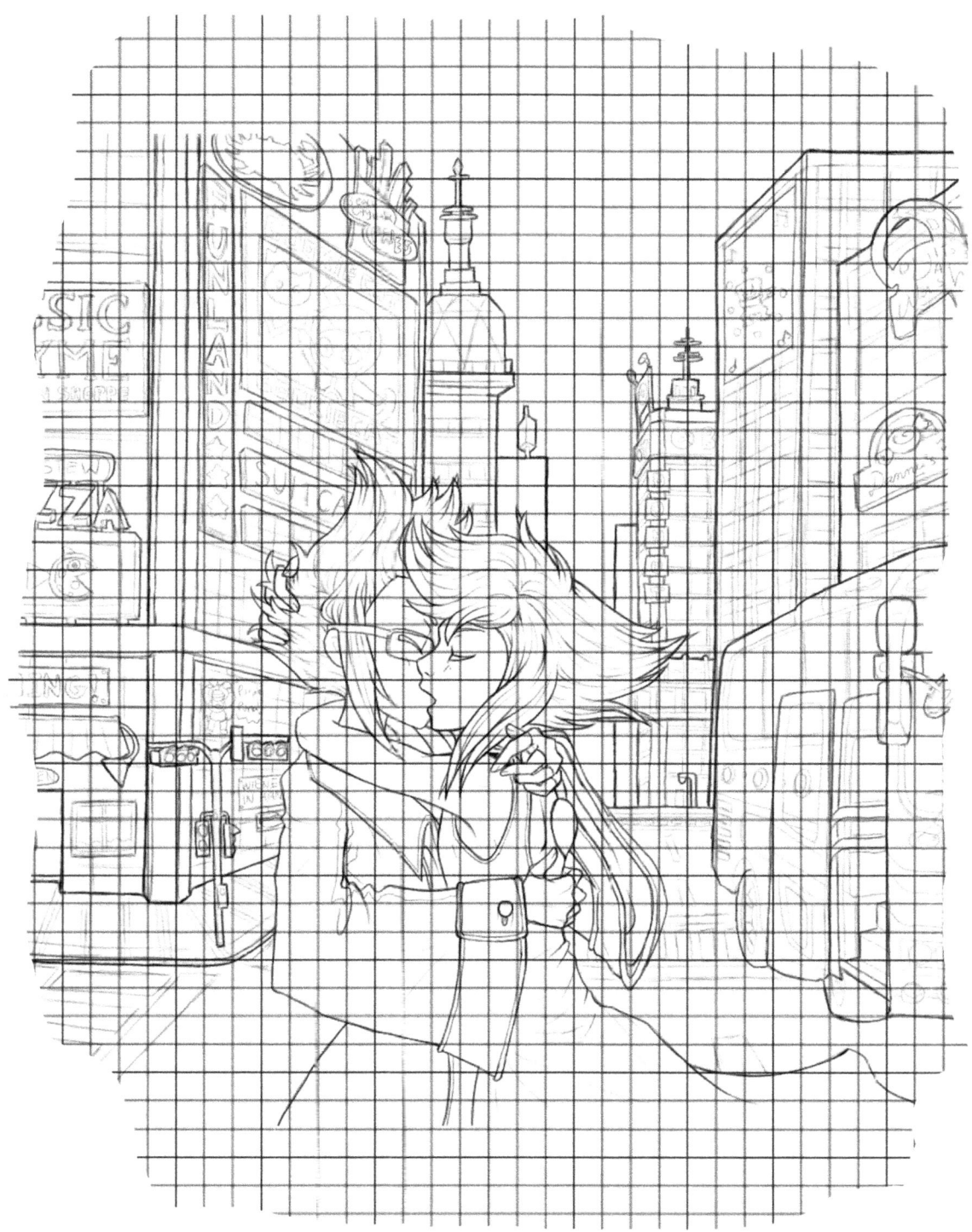

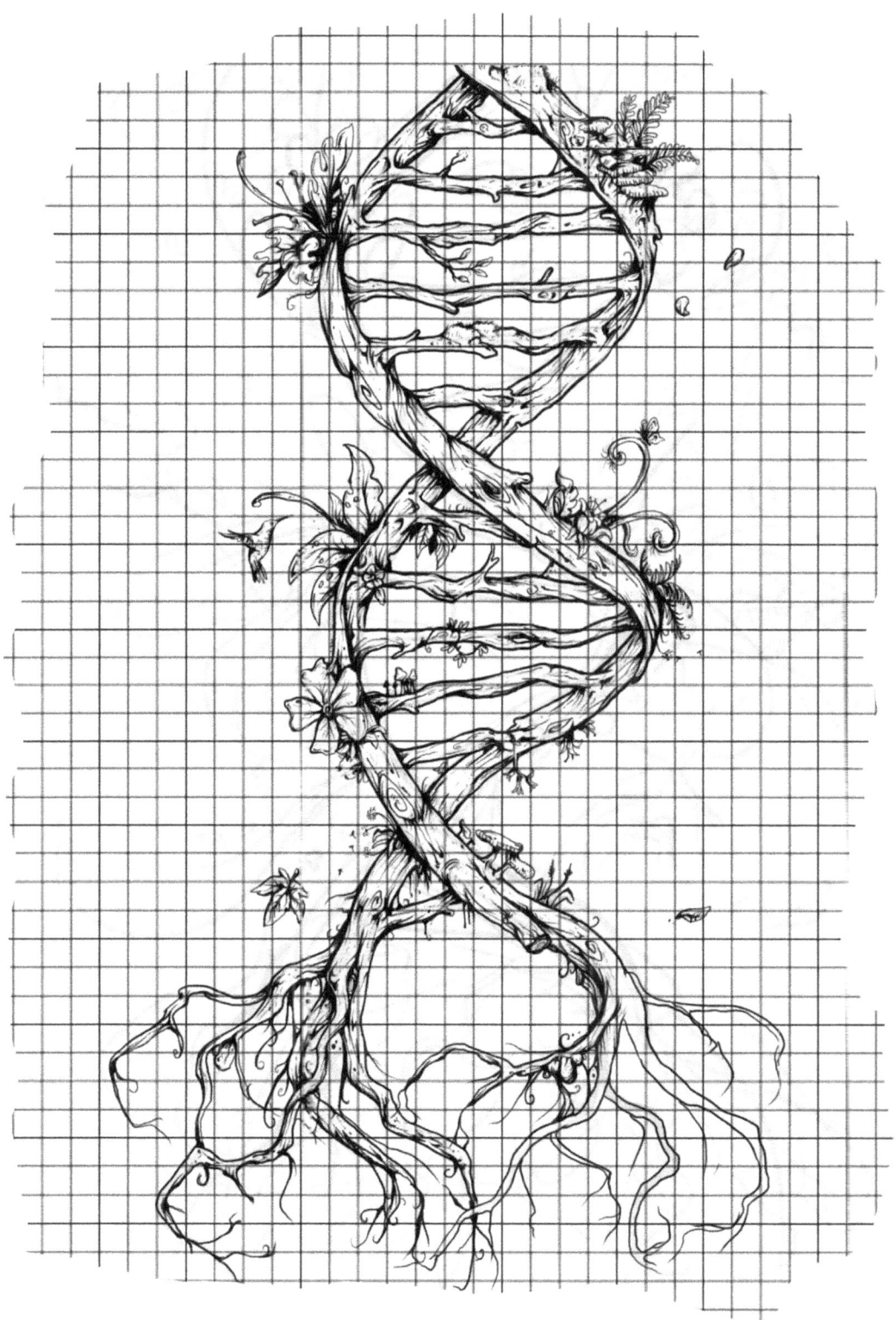

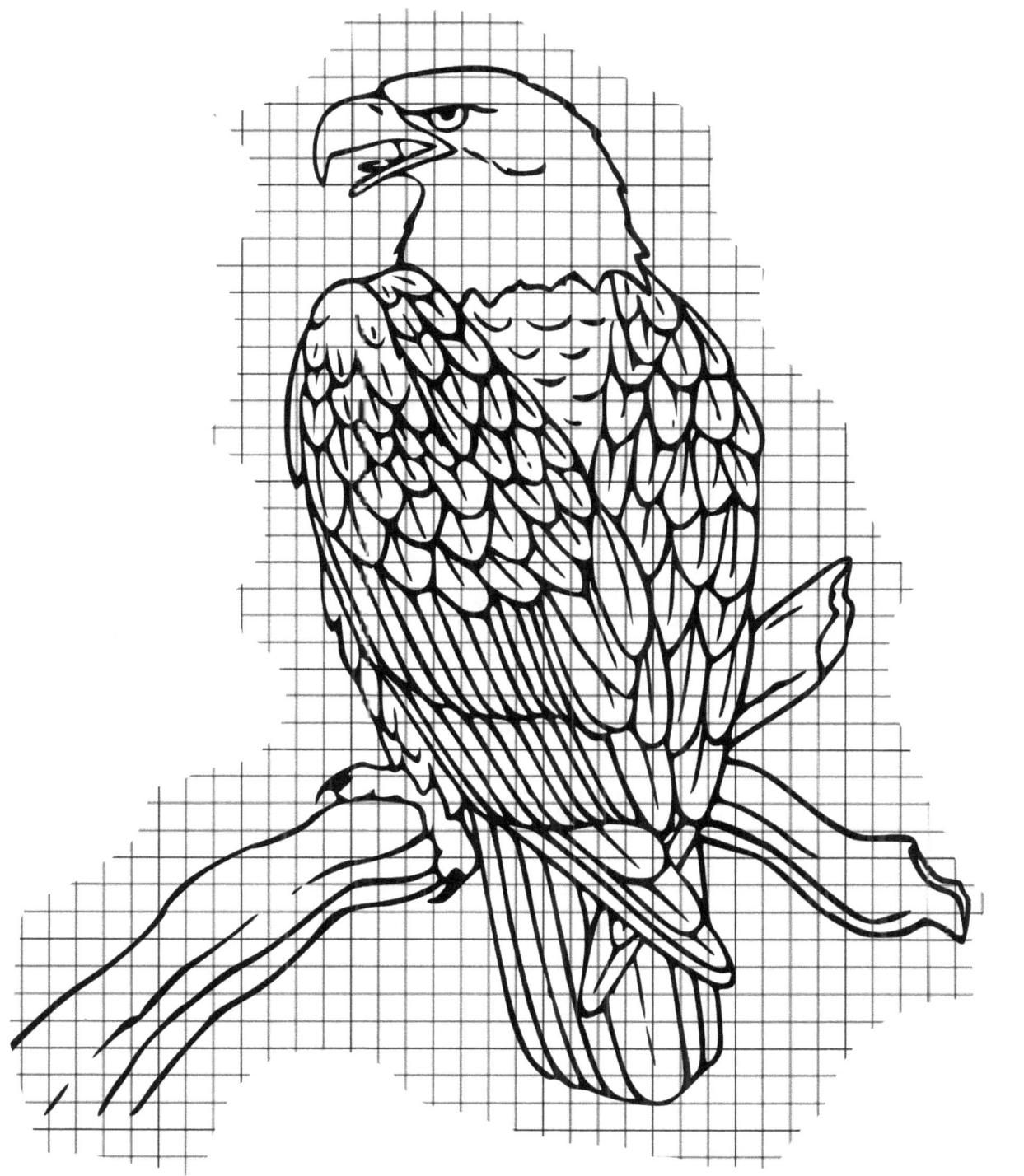

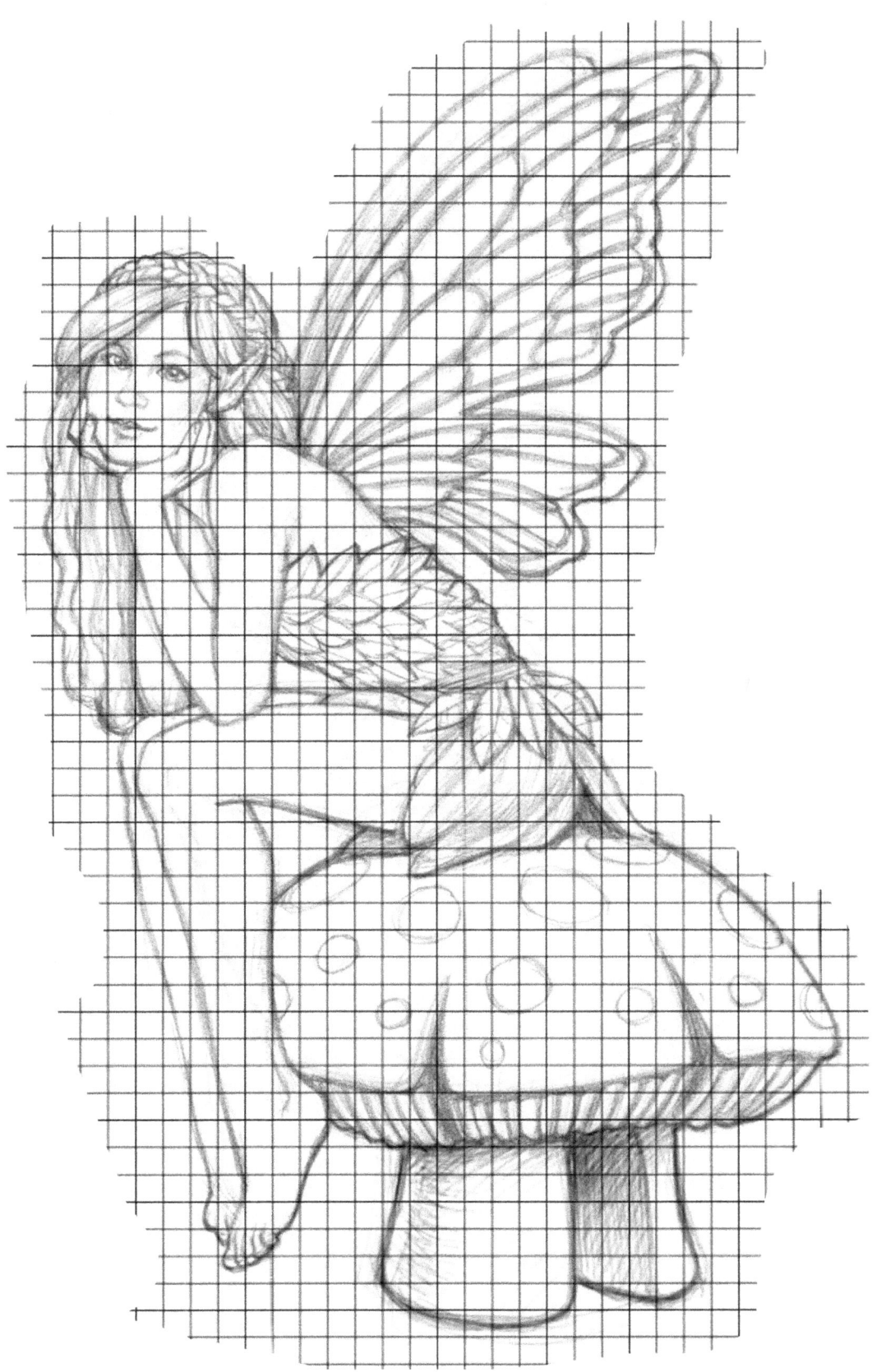

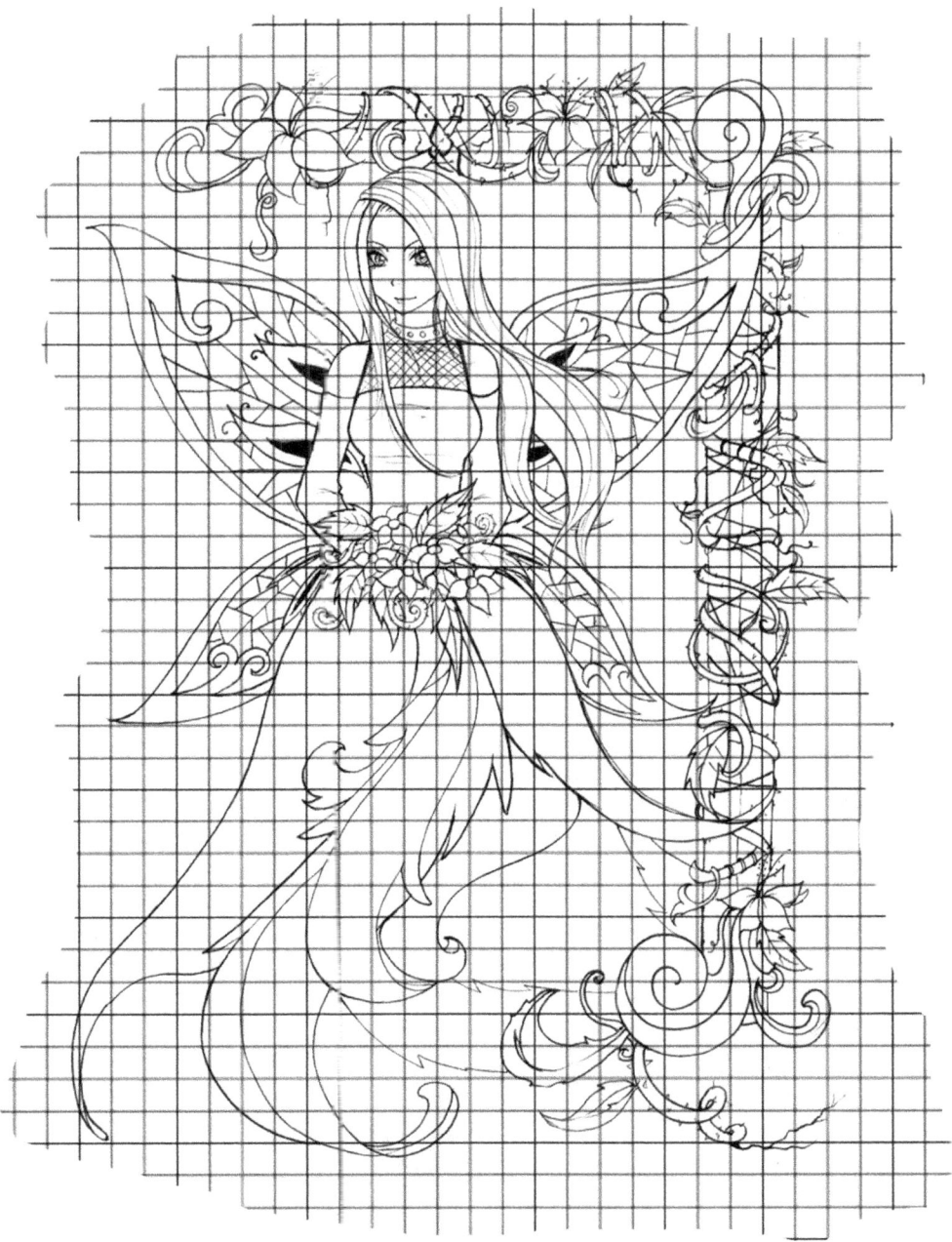

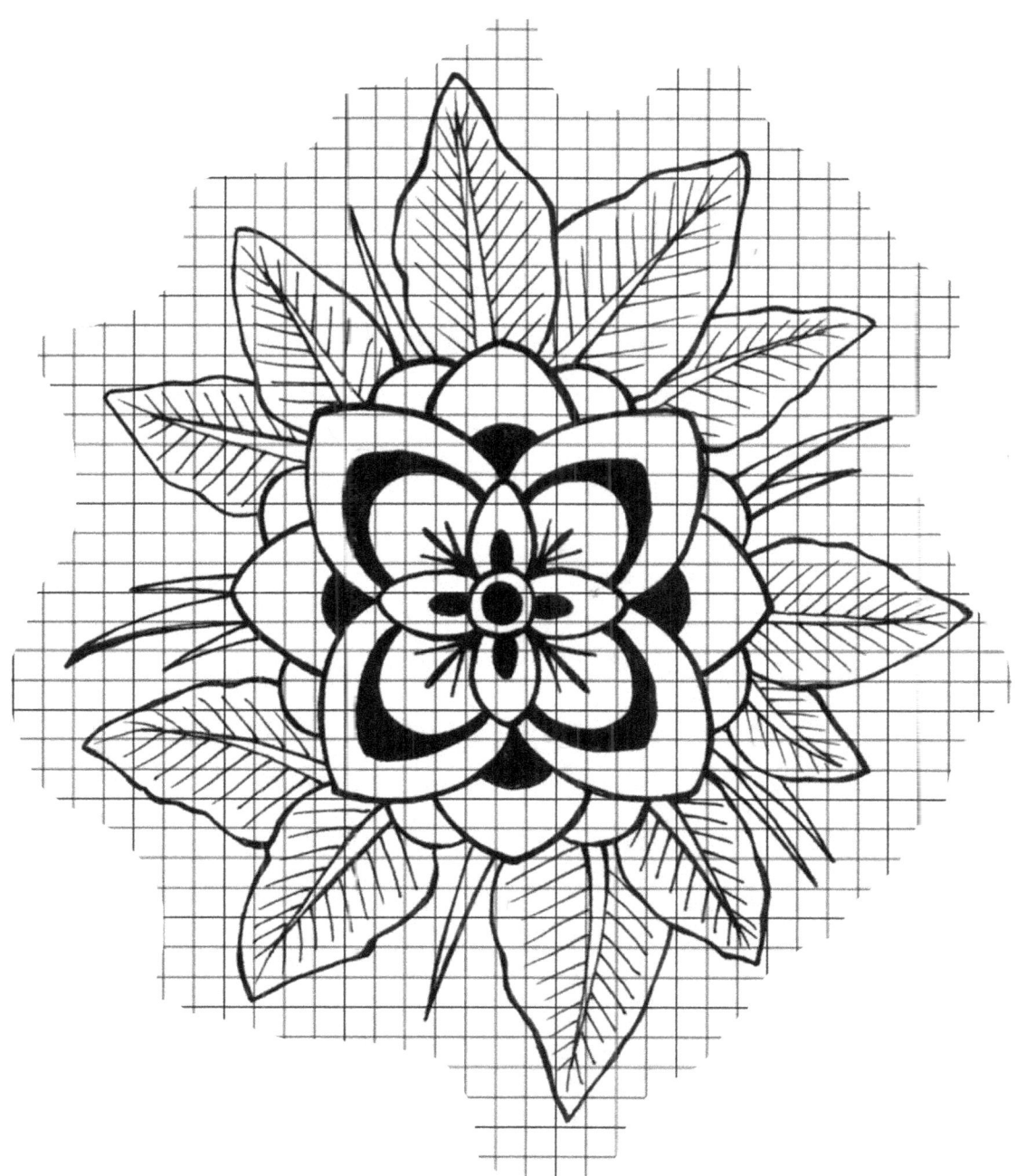

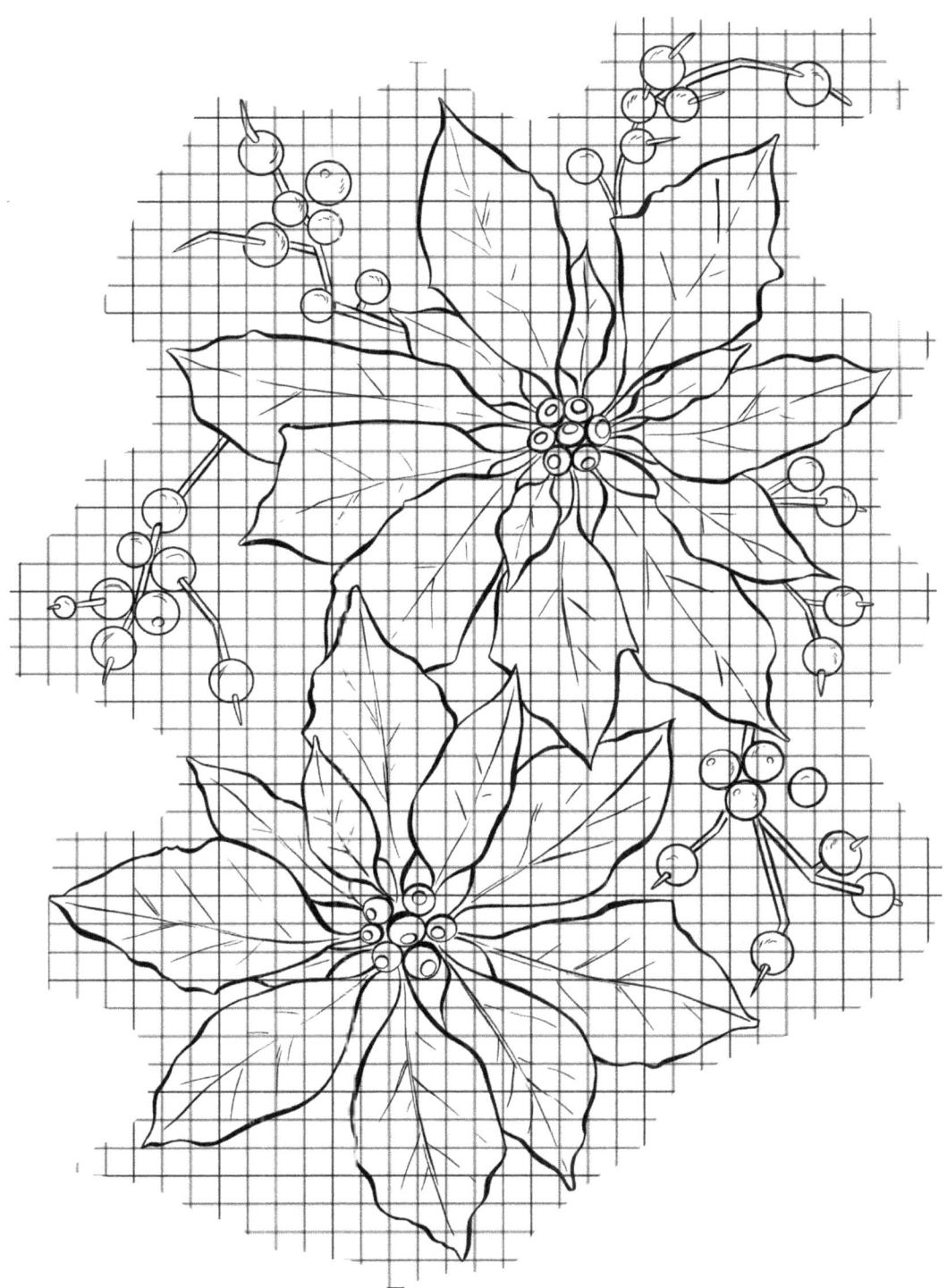

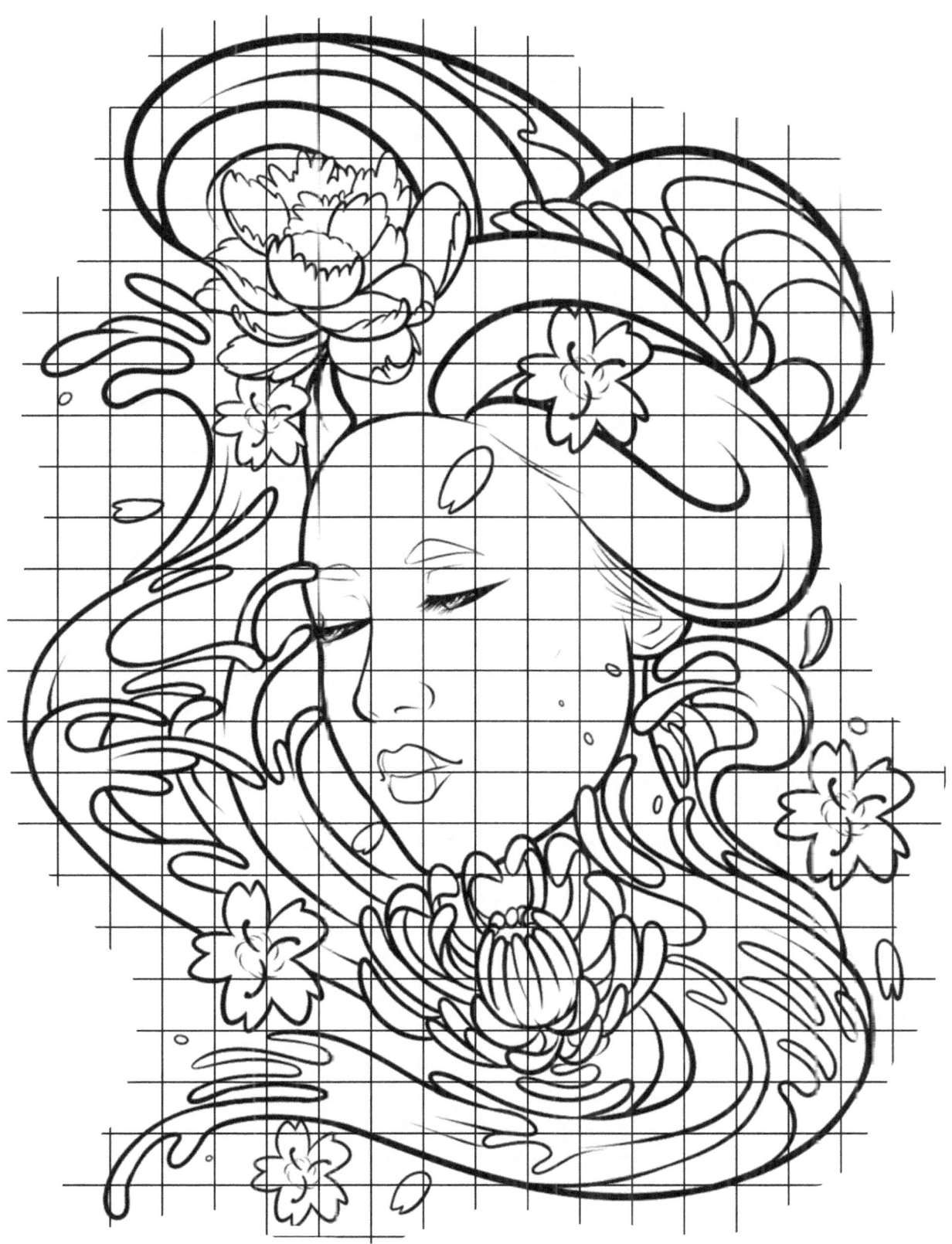

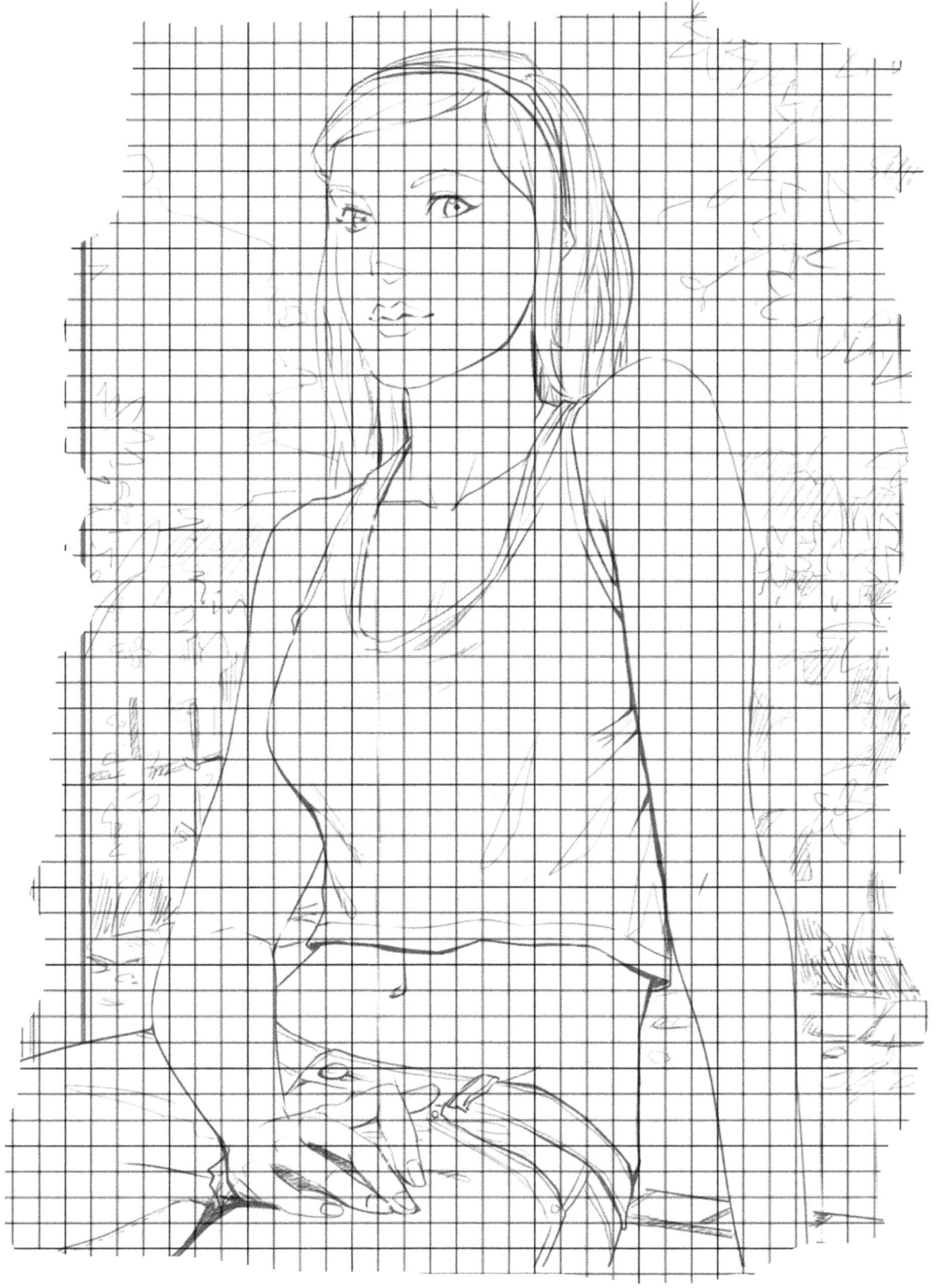

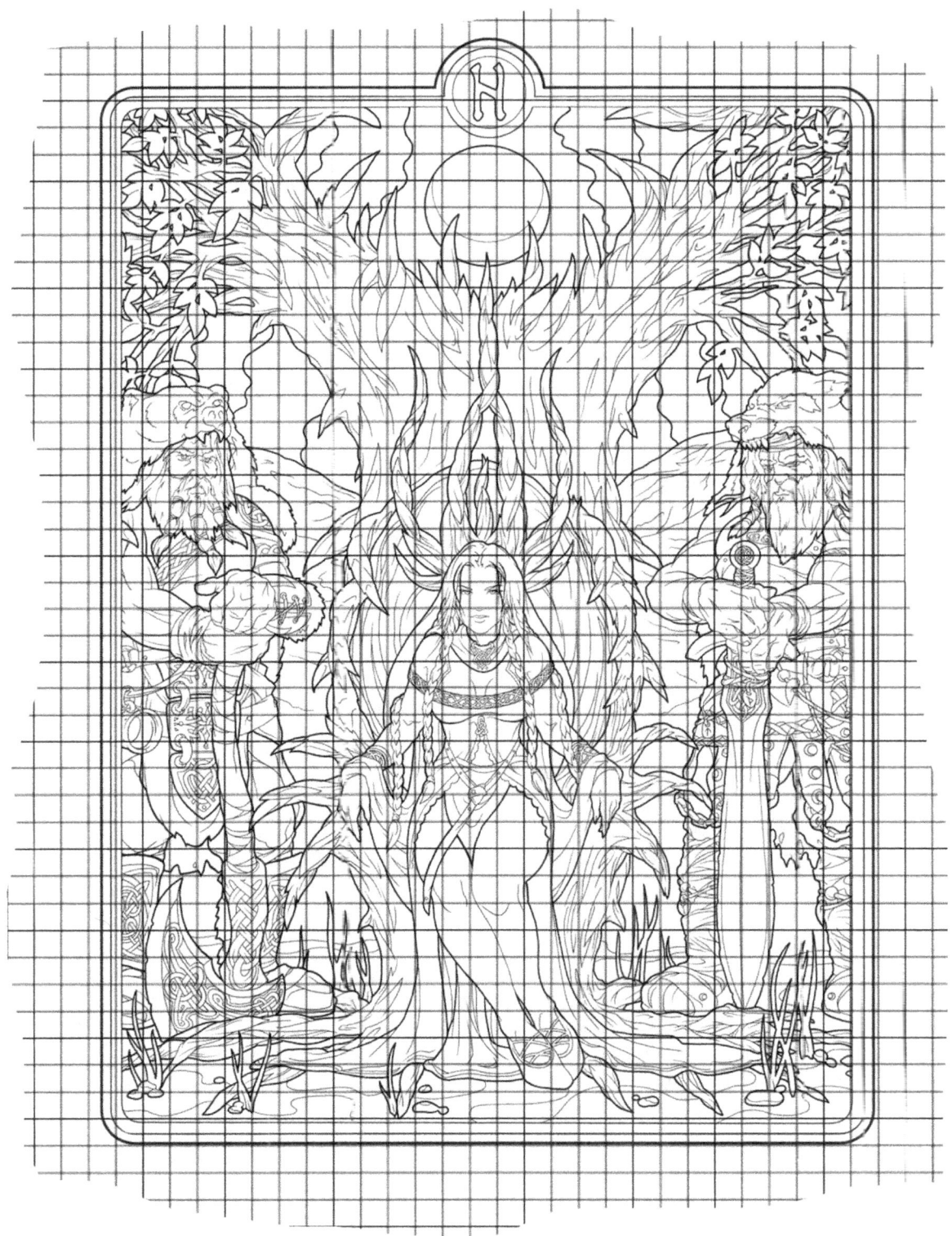

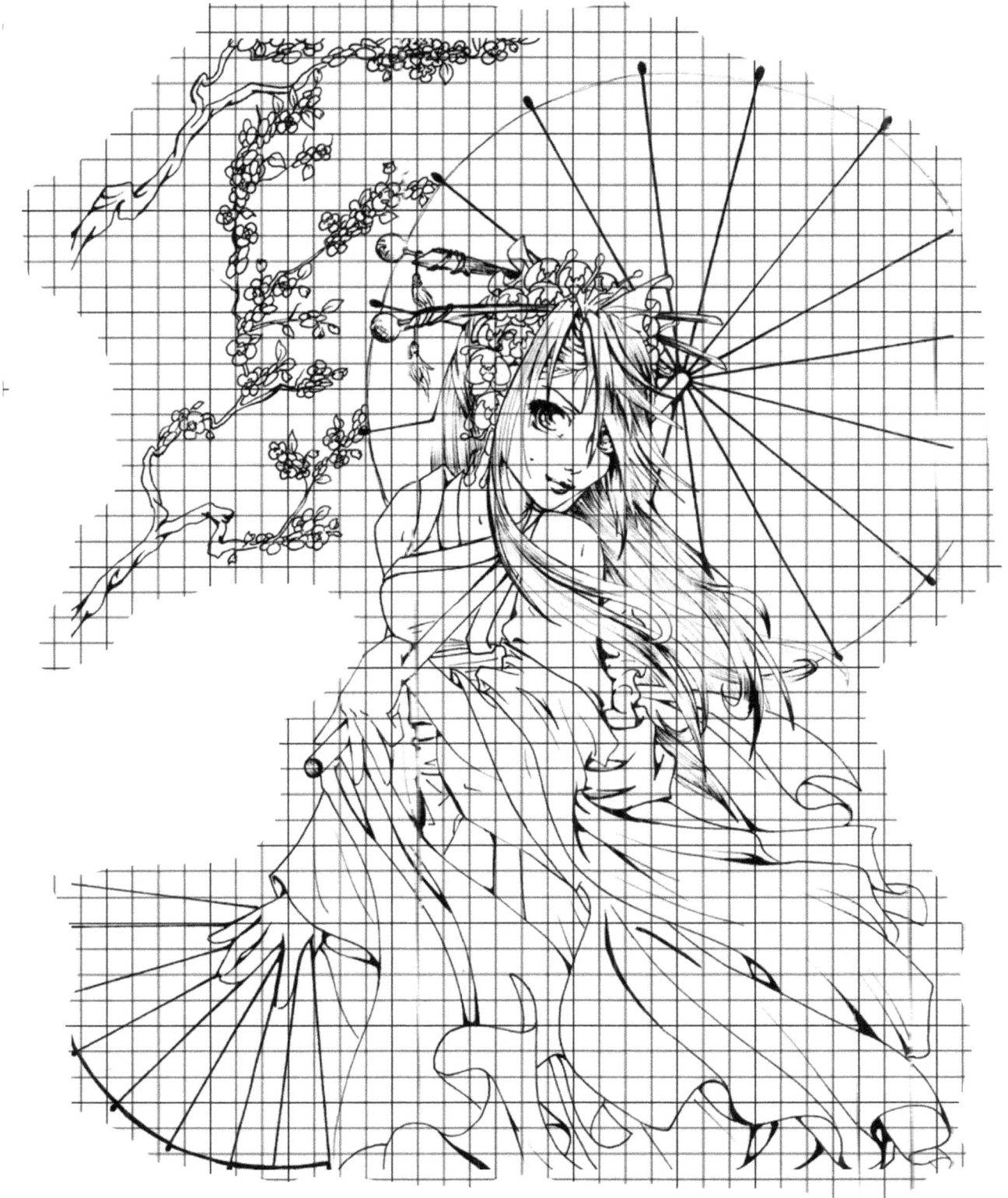

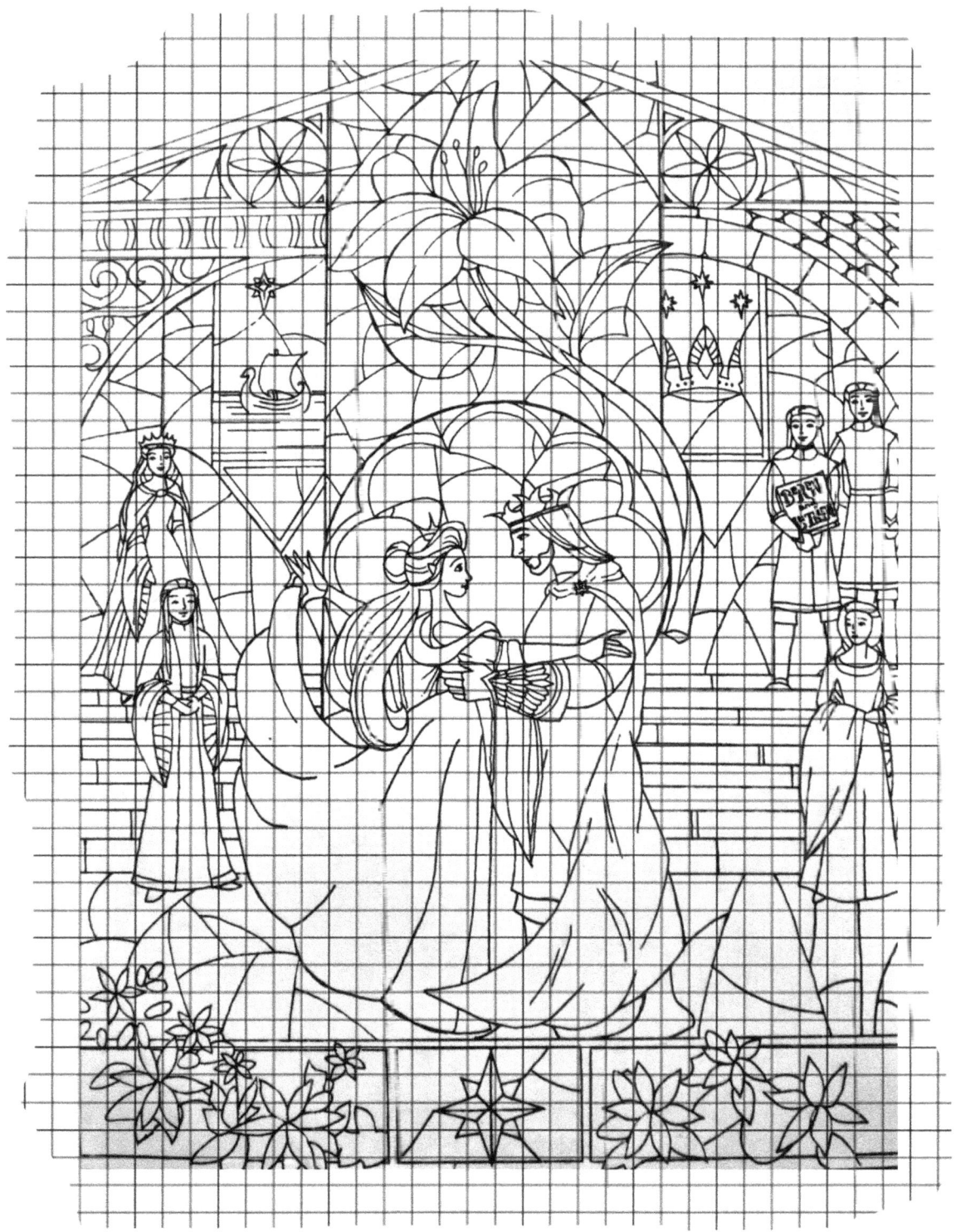

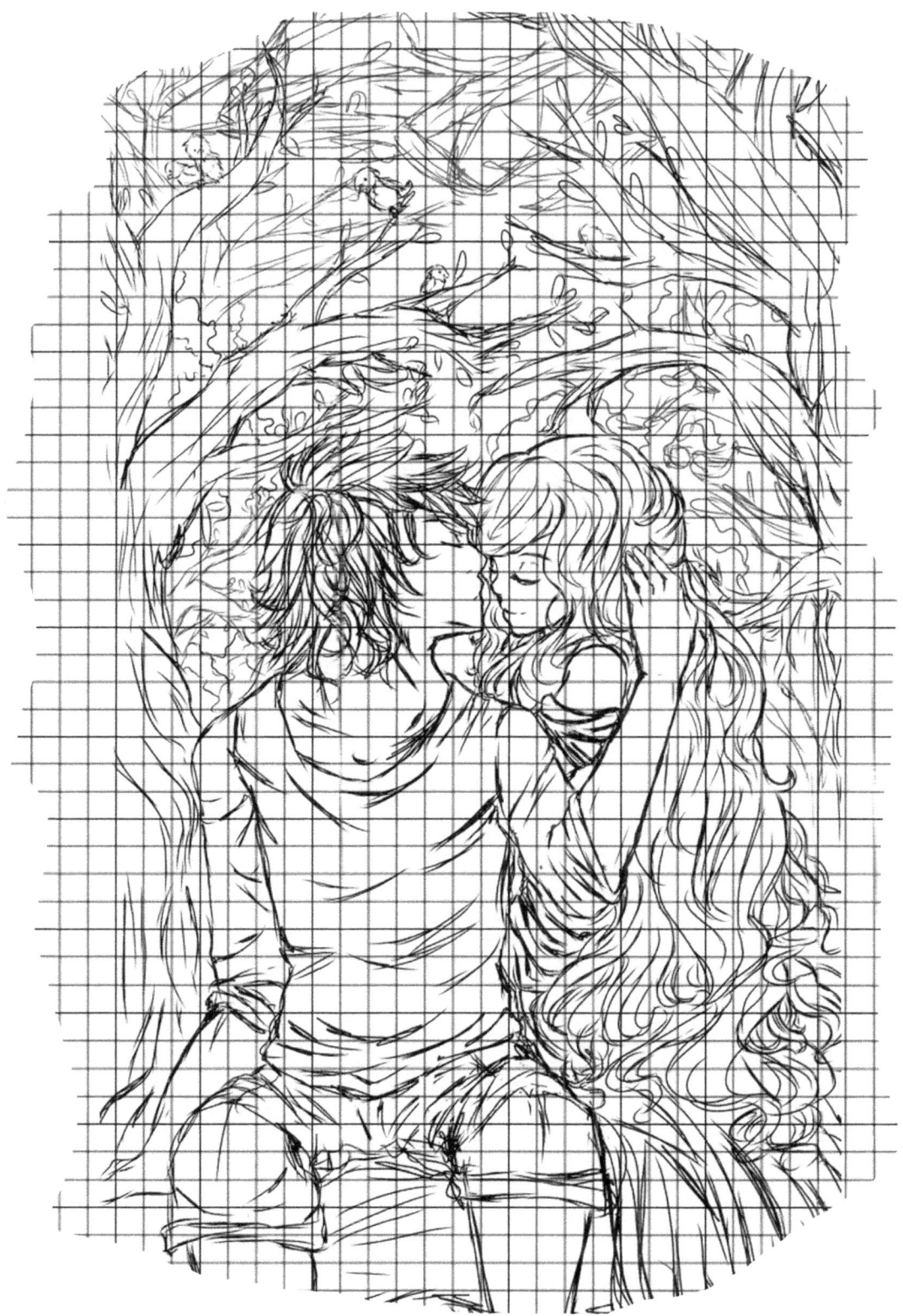

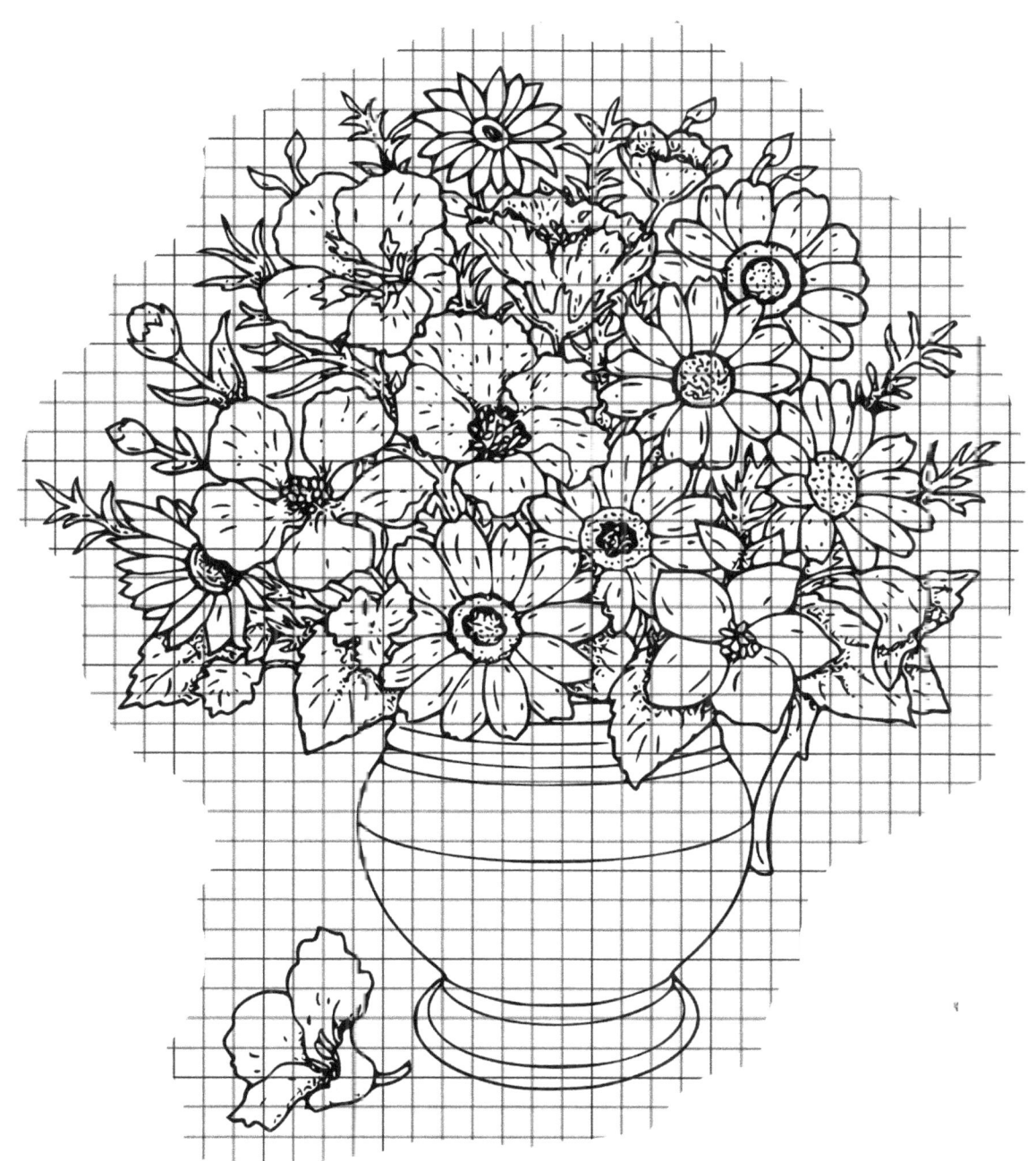

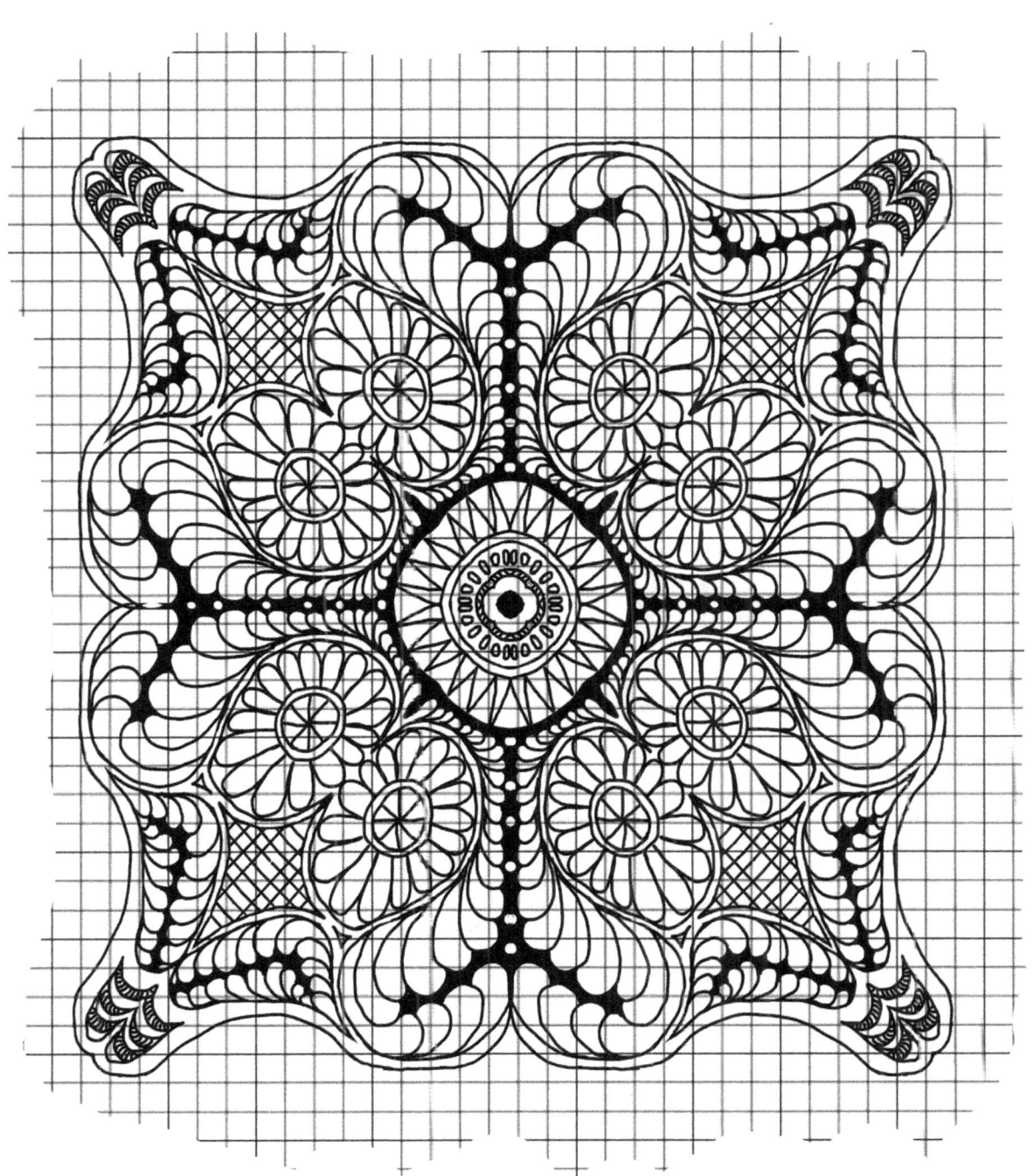

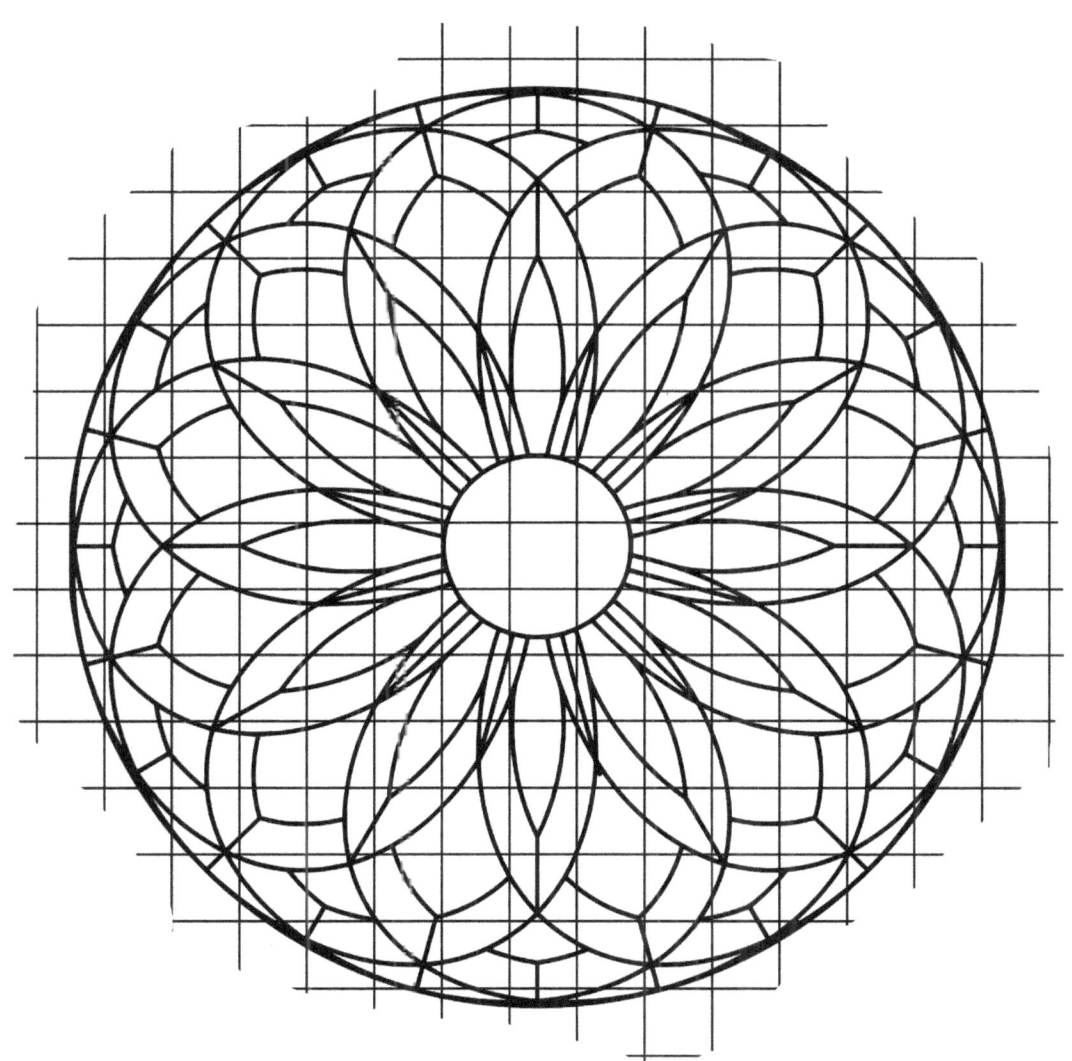

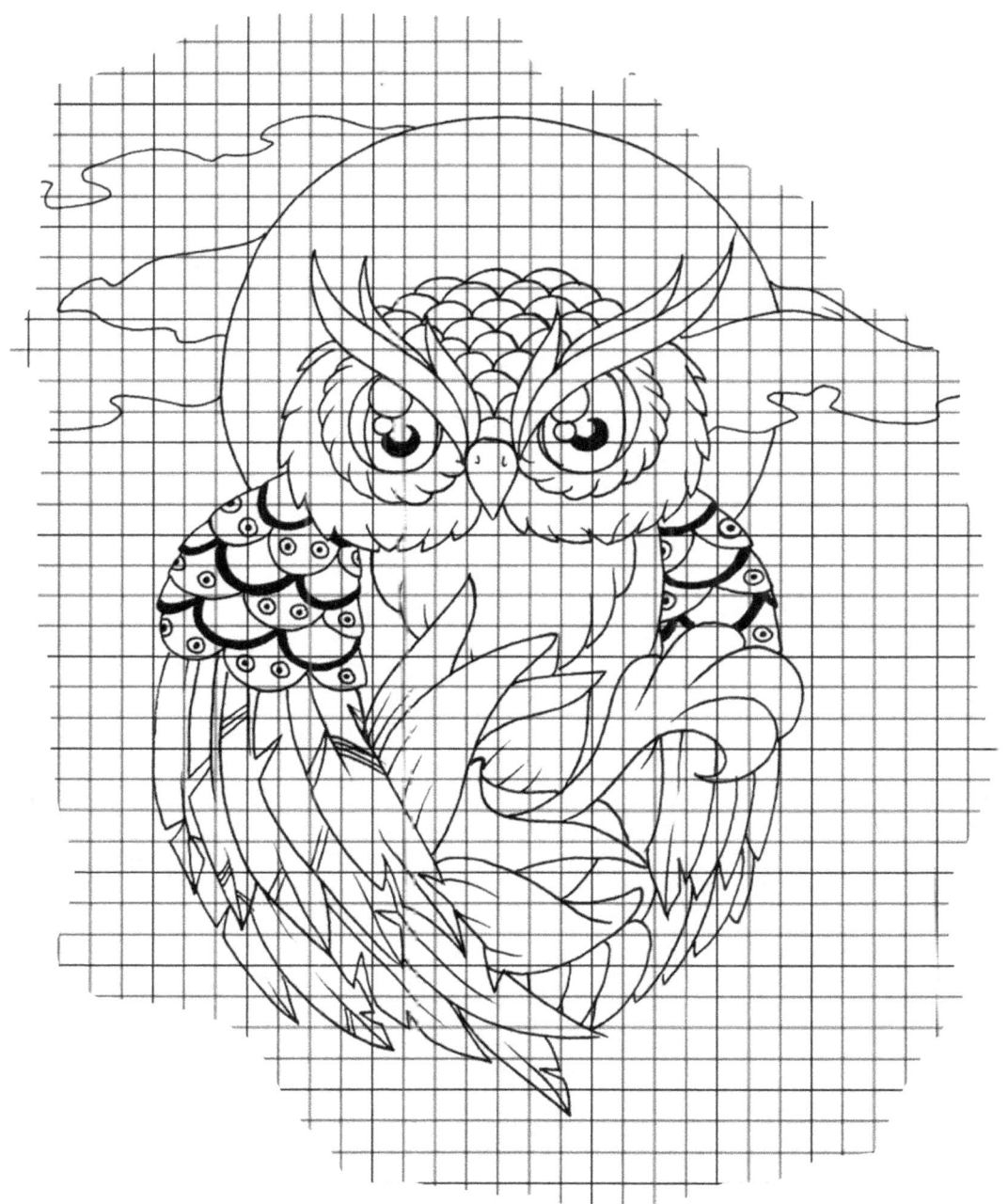

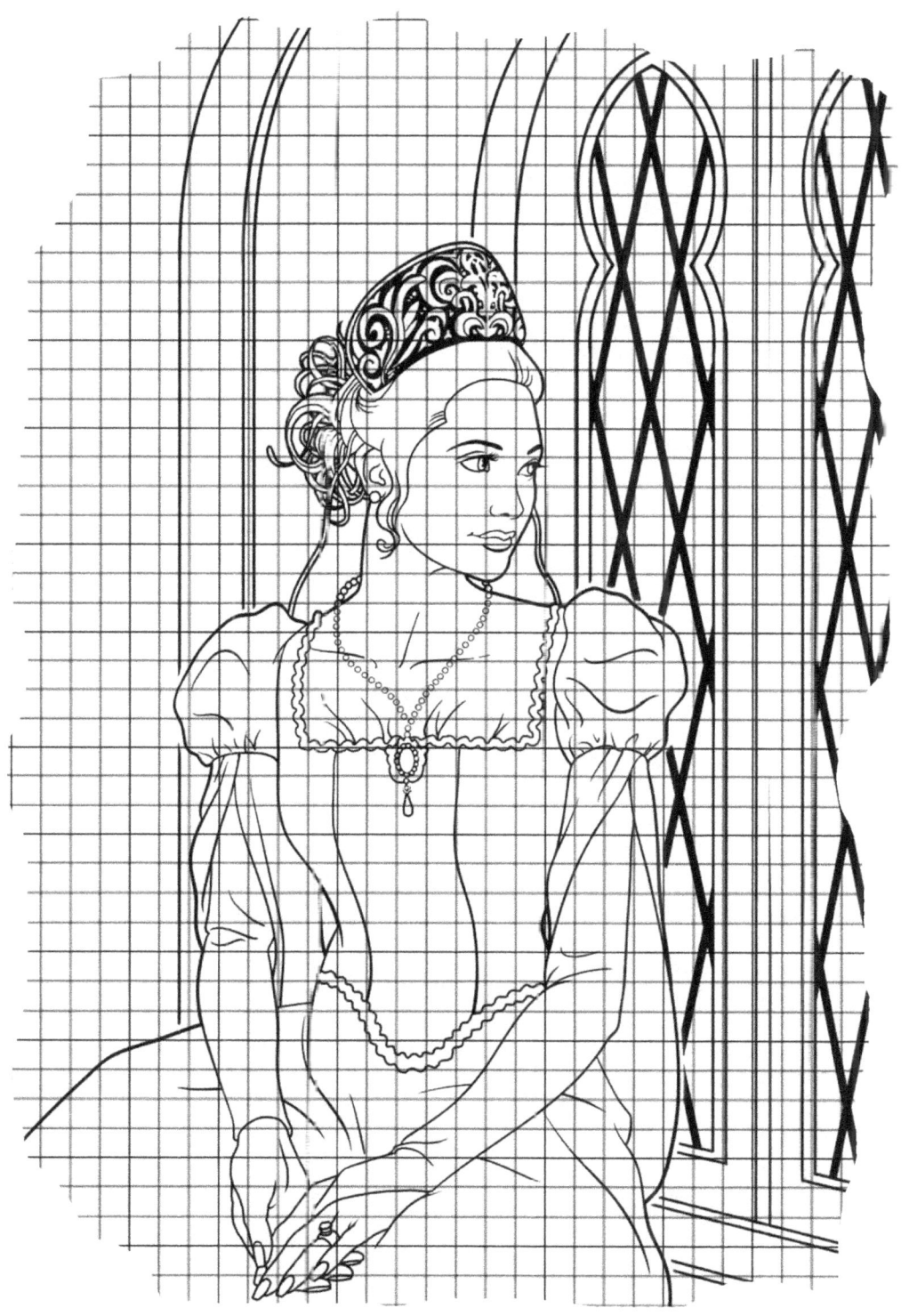

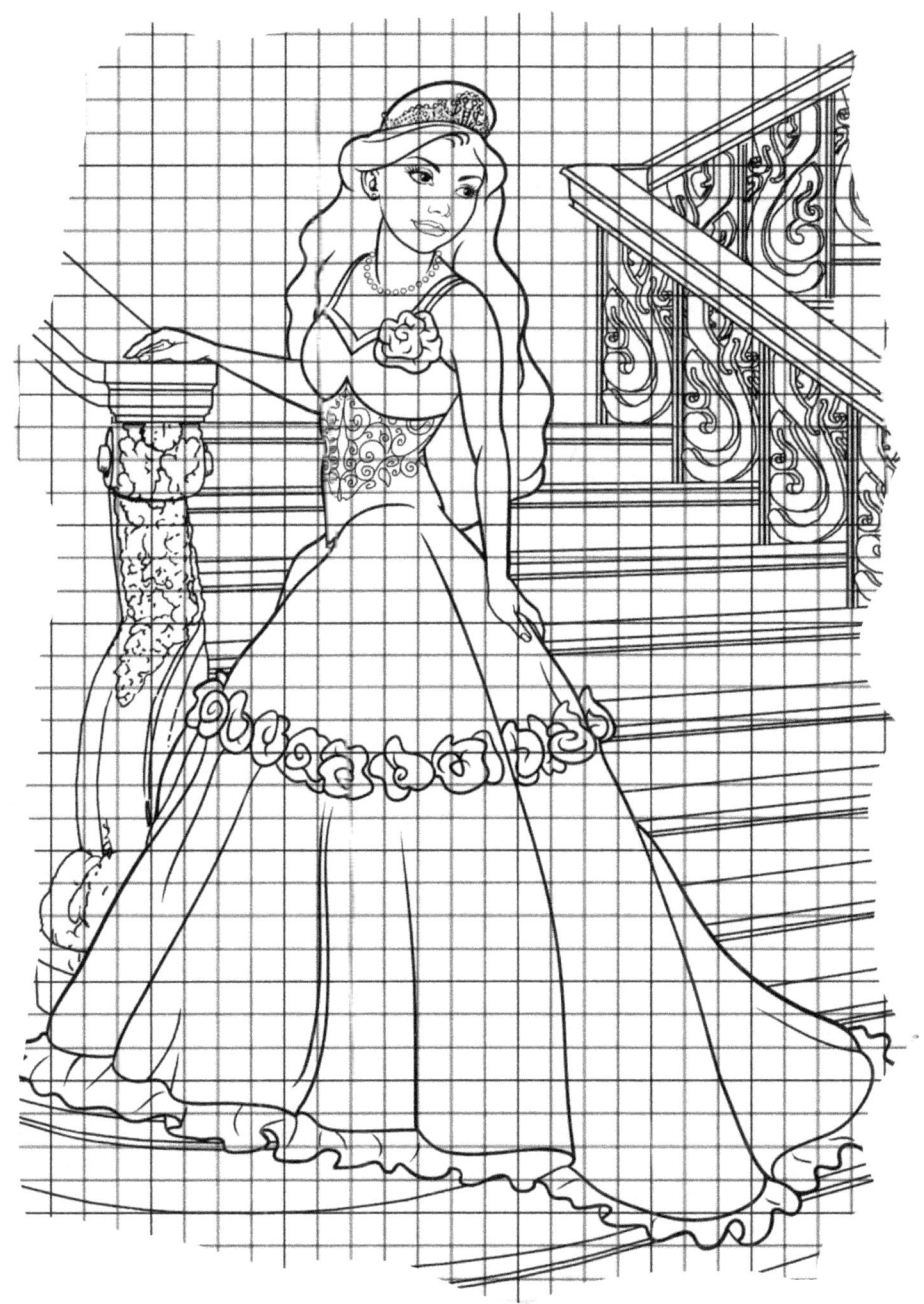

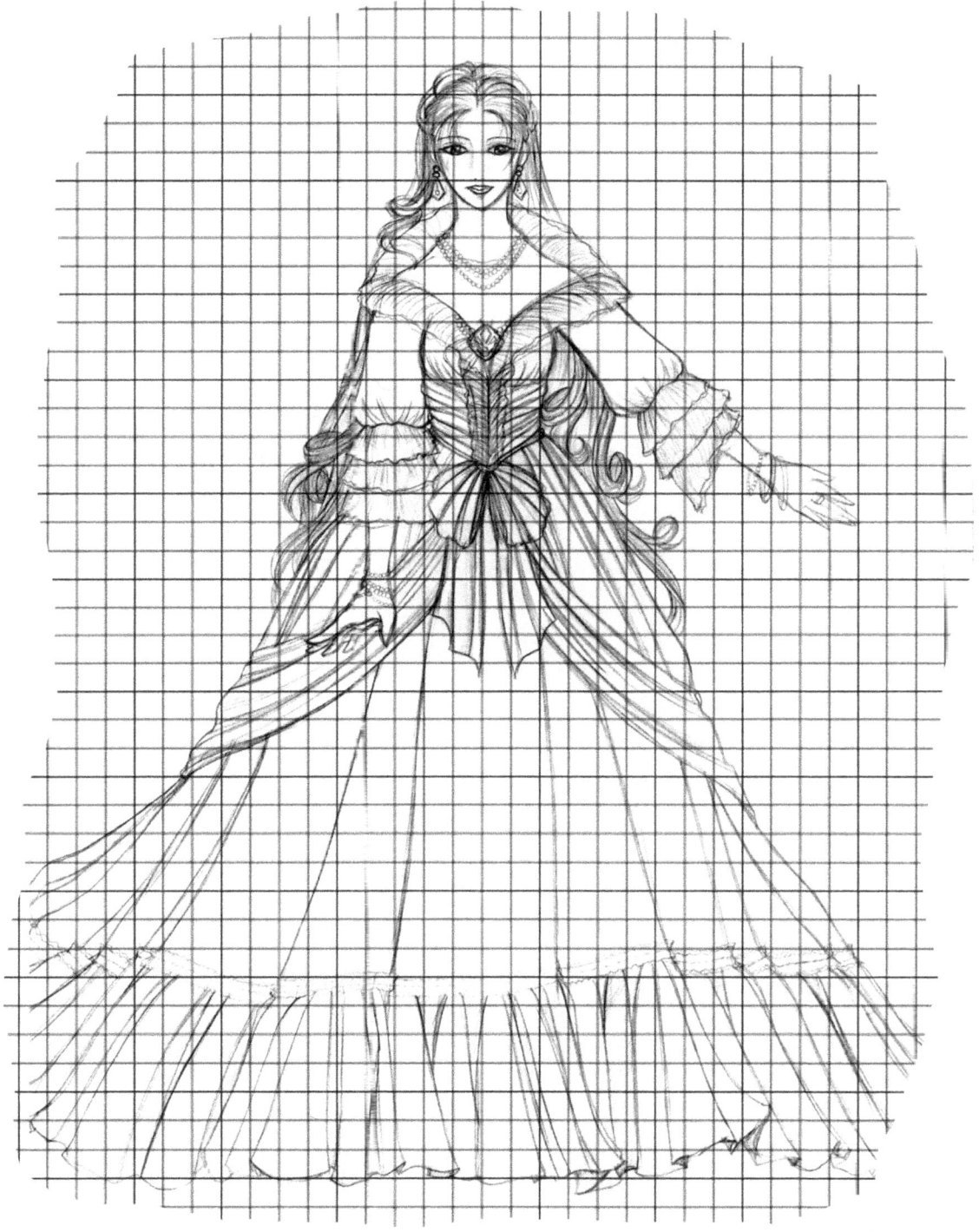

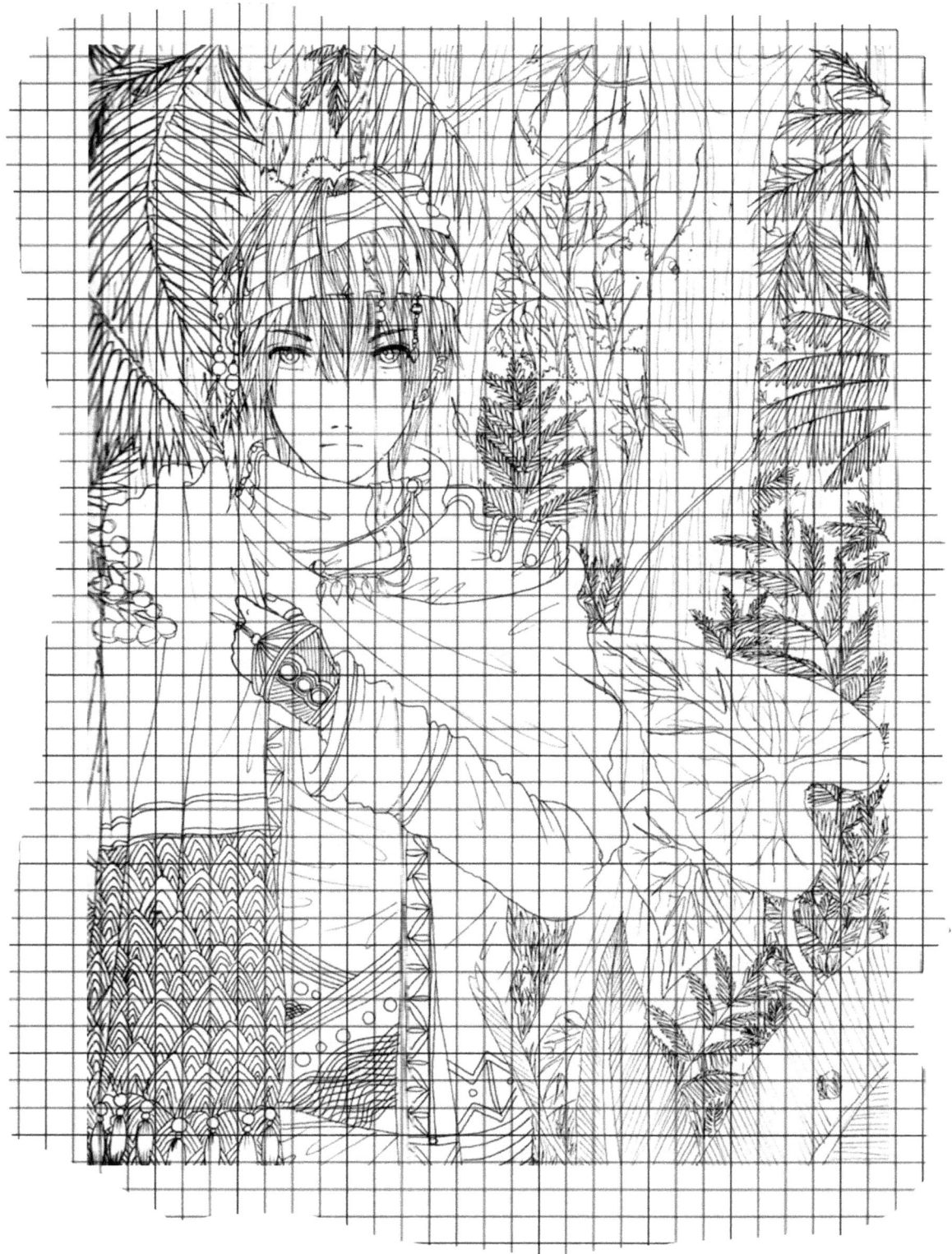

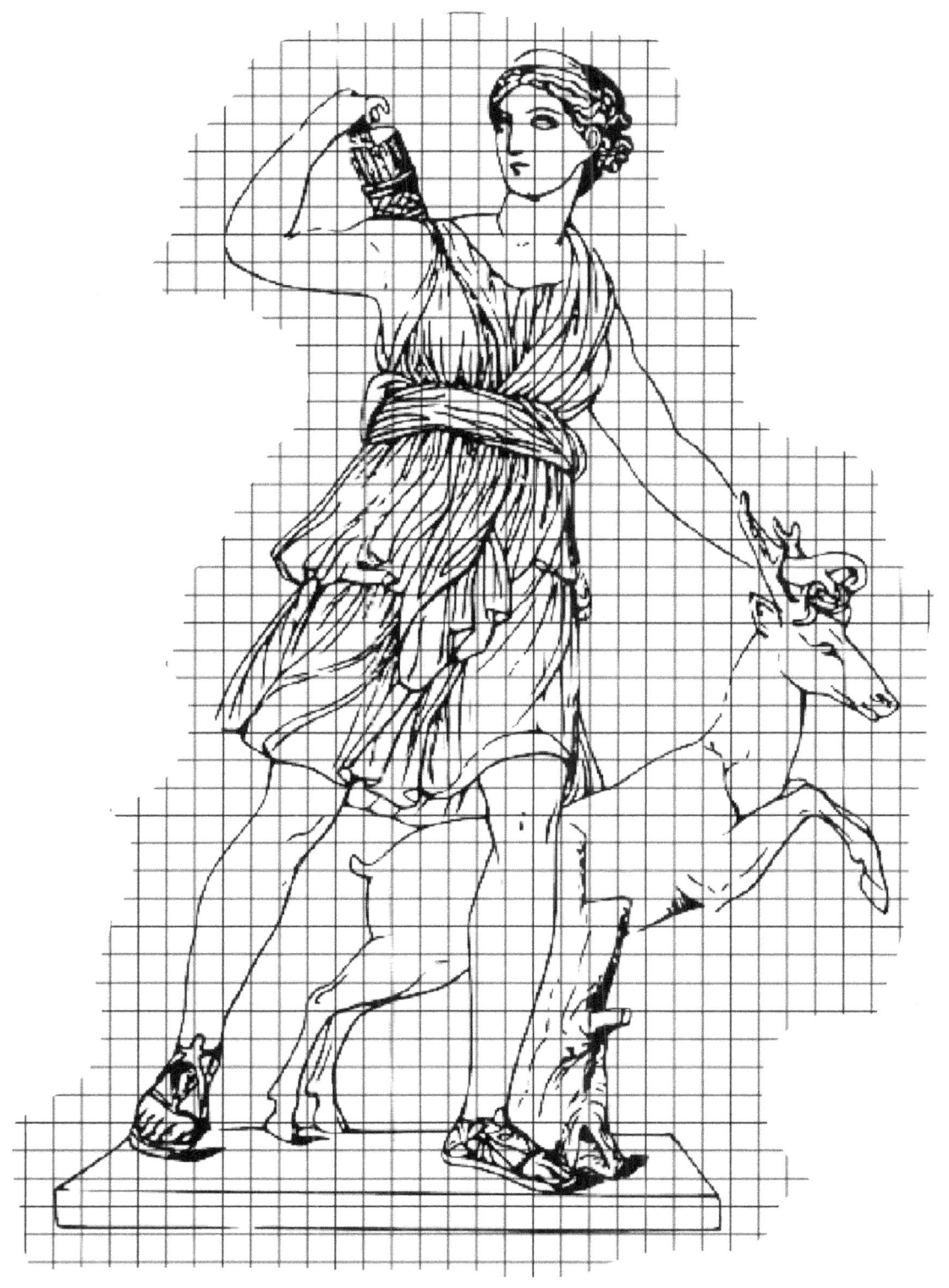

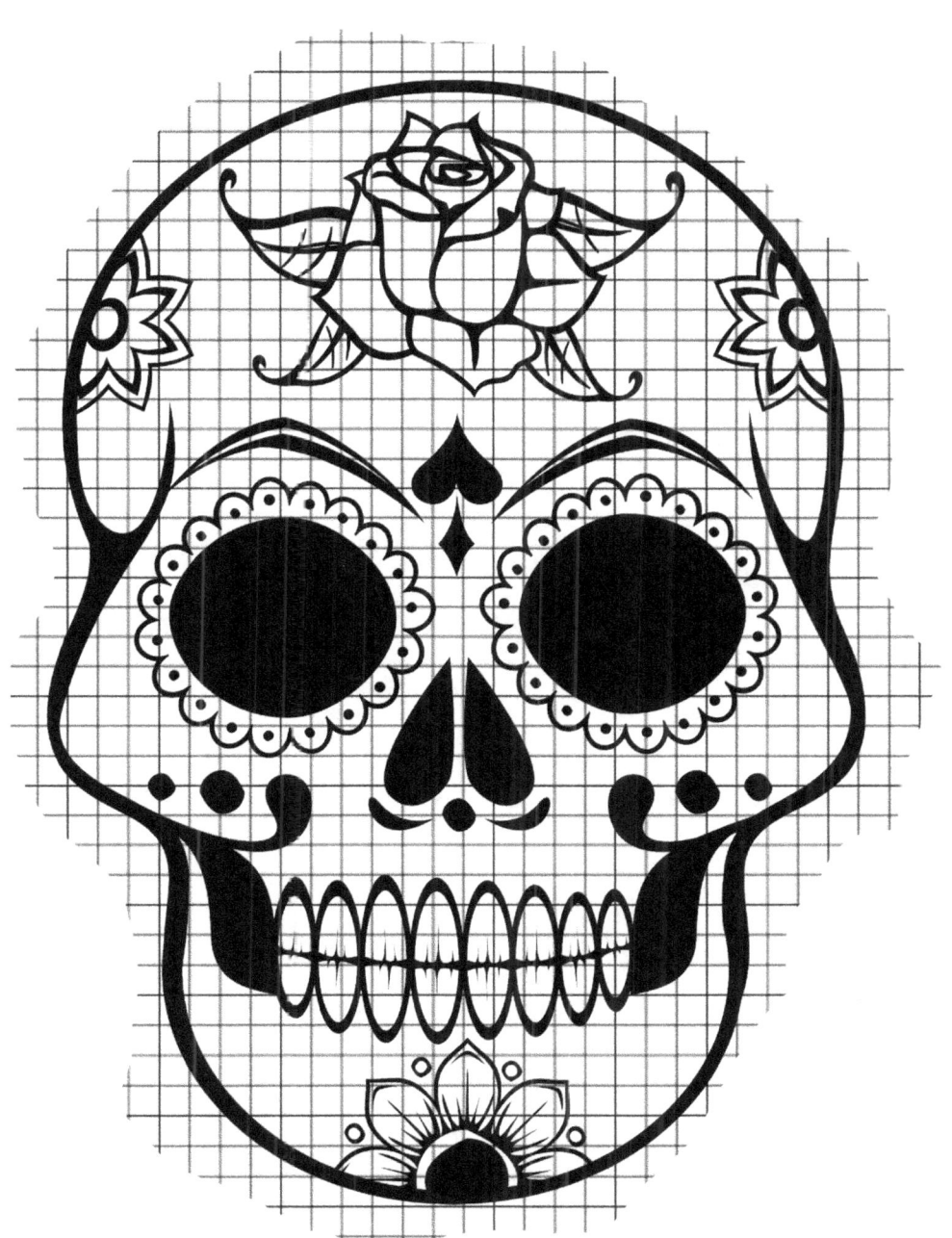

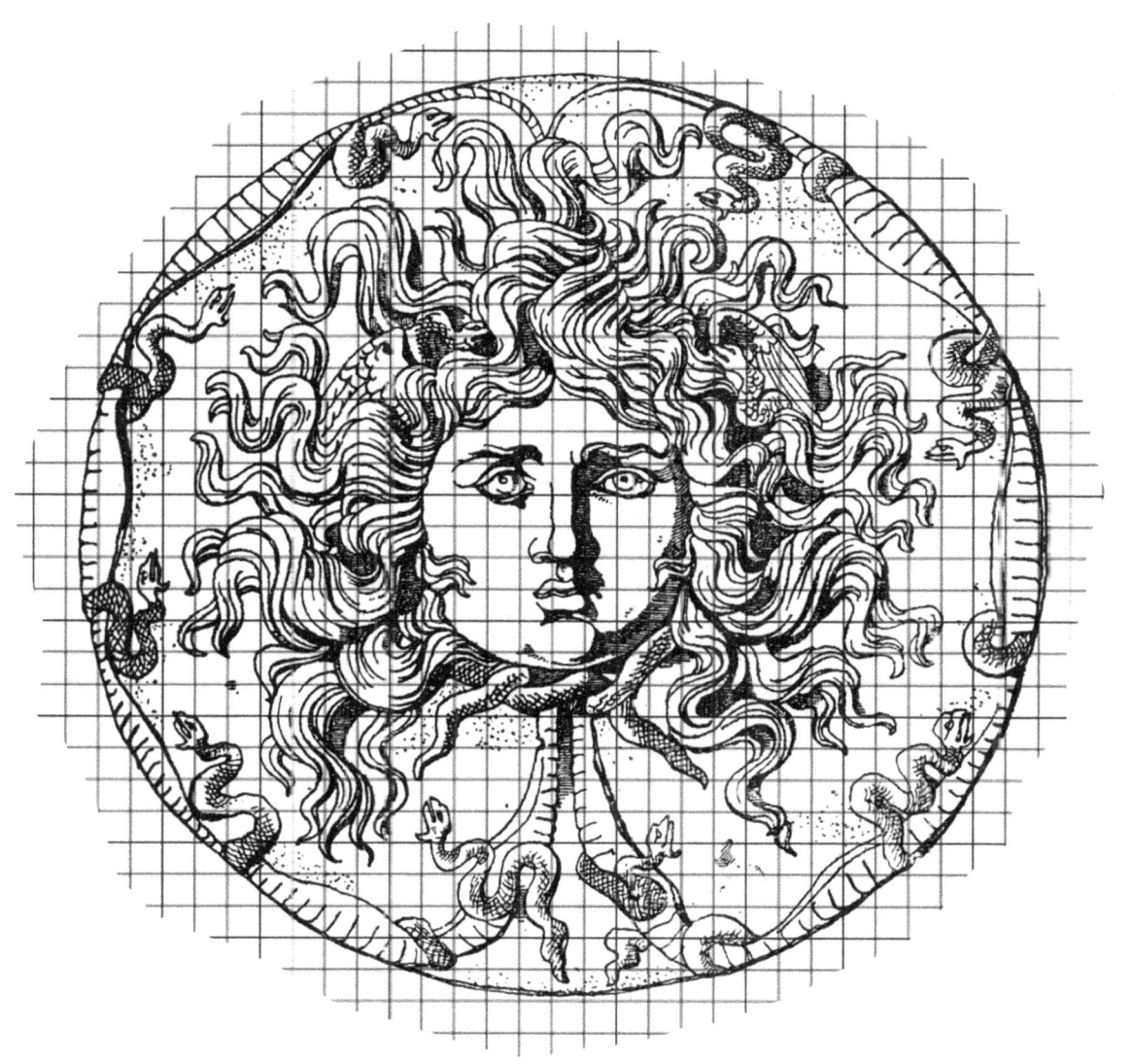

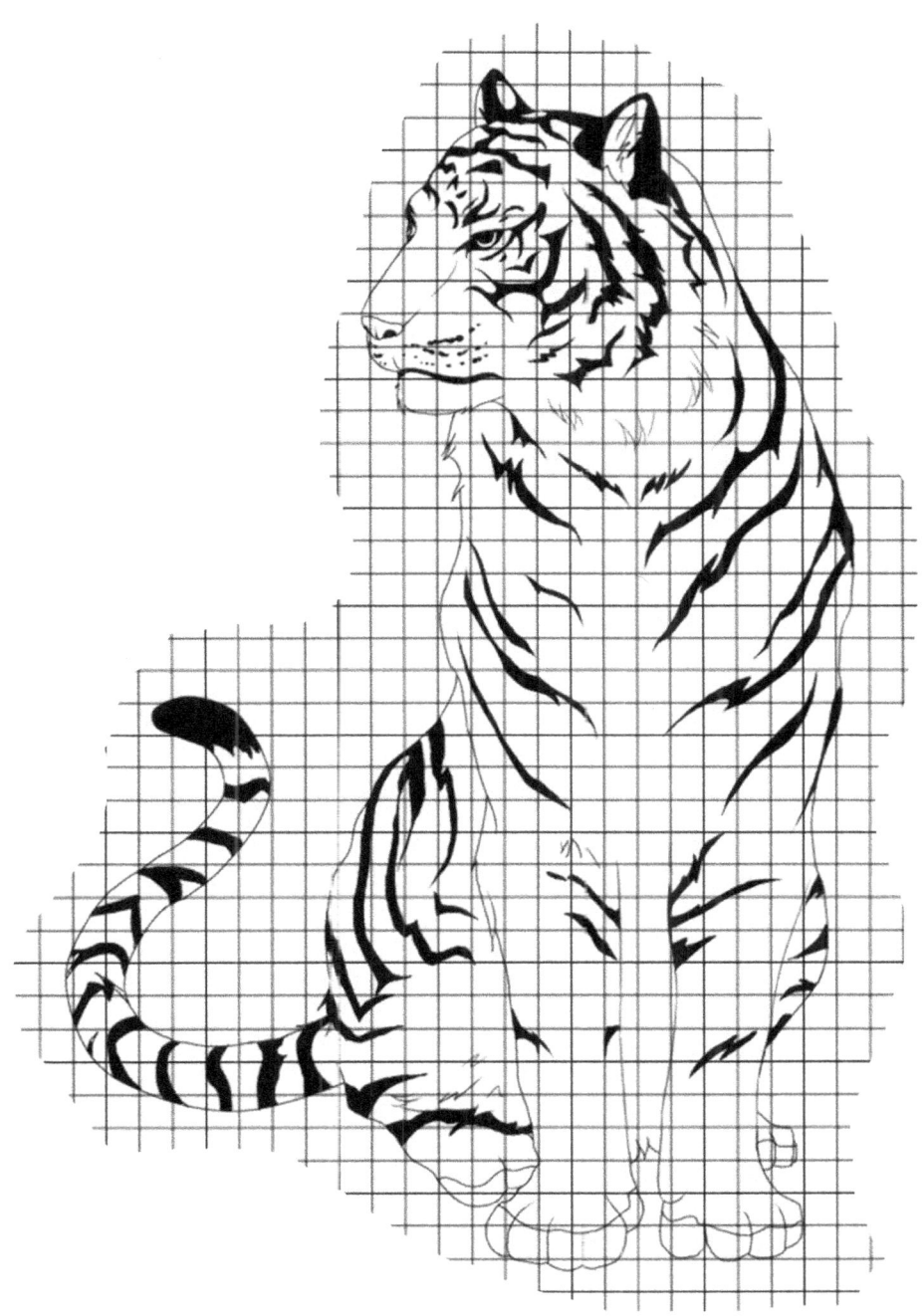

www.jamesdouglaslayton.com

...to get some freebies or just see what else I do.

or

...scan this with your phone to win a free book!!

"Calm down and color"

James Douglas Layton
10 Lyndon Croft
B37 7EW
United Kingdom